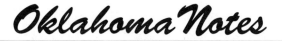

Oklahoma Notes

Clinical Sciences Review for Medical Licensure
Developed at
The University of Oklahoma College of Medicine

Ronald S. Krug, *Series Editor*

Suitable Reviews for:
United States Medical Licensing Examination
(USMLE), Step 2
Federation Licensing Examination (FLEX)

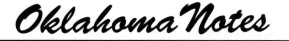

Oklahoma Notes

General Surgery

M. Alex Jacocks

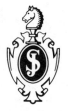

Springer-Verlag
New York Berlin Heidelberg London Paris
Tokyo Hong Kong Barcelona Budapest

M. Alex Jacocks, M.D.
Department of Surgery
College of Medicine
Health Sciences Center
The University of Oklahoma
Oklahoma City, OK 73190
USA

Library of Congress Cataloging-in-Publication Data
Jacocks, M. Alex.
    General surgery / M. Alex Jacocks.
        p.   cm. — (Oklahoma notes)
        ISBN 0-387-97958-1. — ISBN 3-540-97958-1
        1. Surgery—Outlines, syllabi, etc.   I. Title.   II. Series.
        [DNLM: 1. Surgery—outlines.   WO 18 J17p]
    RD37.3.J3   1993
    617.9—dc20
    DNLM/DLC
    for Library of Congress   92-48929

Printed on acid-free paper.

Production managed by Jim Harbison; manufacturing supervised by Jacqui Ashri.
Camera-ready copy prepared by the author.
Printed and bound by Edwards Brothers, Inc., Ann Arbor, MI.
Printed in the United States of America.

9 8 7 6 5 4 3

ISBN 0-387-97958-1 Springer-Verlag New York Berlin Heidelberg
ISBN 3-540-97958-1 Springer-Verlag Berlin Heidelberg New York

Preface to the
Oklahoma Notes

In 1973 the University of Oklahoma College of Medicine instituted a requirement for passage of the Part 1 National Boards for promotion to the third year. To assist students in preparation for this examination a two-week review of the basic sciences was added to the Curriculum in 1975. Ten review texts were written by the faculty. In 1987 these basic science review texts were published as the *Oklahoma Notes* ("Okie Notes") and made available to all students of medicine who were preparing for comprehensive examinations. Over a quarter of a million of these texts have been sold nationally. Their clear, concise outline format has been found to be extremely useful by students preparing themselves for nationally standardized examinations.

Over the past few years numerous inquiries have been made regarding the availability of a Clinical Years series of "Okie Notes." Because of the obvious utility of the basic sciences books, faculty associated with the University of Oklahoma College of Medicine have developed texts in five specialty areas: Medicine, Neurology, Pediatrics, Psychiatry, and Surgery. Each of these texts follows the same condensed outline format as the basic science texts. The faculty who have prepared these texts are clinical educators and therefore the material incorporated in these texts has been validated in the classroom.

Each author has endeavored to distill the "need to know" material from their field of expertise. While preparing these texts, the target audience has always been the clinical years student who is preparing for Step 2 examinations.

A great deal of effort has gone into these texts. I hope they are helpful to you in studying for your licensure examinations.

Ronald S. Krug, Ph.D.
Series Editor

Preface

The material in this text is compiled to help students in the study for board examinations. It is not intended as a textbook, nor is it felt to be a complete reference book. It is my hope that it will be used to jog one's memory of material previously learned and to point out important concepts that should be grasped. The author has made every effort to include the learning objectives as outlined by the Committee on Curriculum of the Association for Surgical Education in this text.

The book is laid out with much the same table of contents as most textbooks in general surgery. It is organized primarily in an organ system fashion but every effort has been made to address common clinical problems and differential diagnoses. It has been written in an outline form and the author would encourage students to highlight important areas, write in the margins, and expand on the concepts or key phrases listed in the book.

M. Alex Jacocks

Acknowledgments

I would like to acknowledge the tremendous amount of work put into this effort by other people on the staff at the University of Oklahoma College of Medicine, in particular, Ms. Judy Wheeler for her tremendous hours at organizing and typing this material and Ms. Sharon Gammill for her expertise with editing.

Contents

Contents

FLUIDS . ELECTROLYTES . NUTRITION

I. Basic principles

    A.   Know what makes up normal body fluid compartments and electrolytes and what sort of maintenance fluid and acid base balance must be done to maintain the normal homeostasis.

    B.   Know what problems are created by common clinical perturbations of the system (i.e., fever, ventilator, biliary fistula, etc.)

    C.   Know the make-up of various commercially available electrolyte solutions and nutritional solutions and how to use them.

II. The normal fluids and electrolytes and their maintenance

    A.   Fluid requirements

        1.   Normal adult male is 60% body water by weight.

            a.   40% is intracellular - 20% extracellular (16% interstitial and 4% intravascular).

            b.   Maintenance of body water largely controlled by release of antidiuretic hormone from the posterior pituitary to increase tubular water resorption in the kidney and aldosterone secretion from the adrenal gland to retain sodium and water in a more passive fashion.

2.   Common replacement formula

> 0 - 10 kg body weight - replace 100 cc/kg/24 hr
> 10 - 30 kg body weight - replace 50 cc/kg/24 hr
> \> 30 kg body weight - replace 20 cc/kg/24 hr

    a.   Example: 70 kg man gets 1000 cc's for his first 10 kg of body weight, 1000 cc's for the next 20 kg of body weight, and 800 cc's for the next 40 kg of body weight. If this is given equally over 24 hours, a rate of 125 cc's per hour would be used.

3.   Assessment of fluid status

    a.   Physical exam - pulse, blood pressure, skin turgor, mental activity, etc.

    b.   Urine output - expect 0.5 cc/kg/hour in adults; 1-2 cc/kg/hour in infants and children.

    c.   Careful record of input and output.

    d.   Invasive monitoring using a central venous pressure line or pulmonary capillary wedge pressure with a Swan-Ganz catheter.

    e.   Daily weights - for overall long-term management.

4.   Normal losses

    a.   Urine - most patients lose approximately 1500 cc's of urine per day.

    b.   Feces - approximately 200-300 cc's of water loss per day in feces.

    c.   Insensible loss - 500-600 cc's of fluid loss per day in insensible losses (pure water).

B.   Electrolytes

1.   Sodium

    a.   Is the most common extracellular cation with normal concentration of 135-145 mEq/liter in the serum.

    b.   Total body sodium estimated to be 40 mEq/liter which is also the normal replacement value of fluids for normal maintenance.

      c.   Sodium resorption in exchange for potassium and hydrogen secretion by the distal renal tubules is the direct effect of aldosterone.

2.   Potassium

      a.   Major intracellular cation with normal serum concentration of 3.5 -5.0 mEq/liter.

      b.   98% of potassium is located intracellularly.

      c.   Potassium excretion is directly related to circulating levels of aldosterone, cellular and extracellular potassium content and tubular urine flow rates. There is a normal loss of potassium of approximately 10-15 mEq/liter in urine which must be replaced.

3.   Chloride

      a.   The major extracellular anion with a normal level of 95-105 mEq/liter.

      b.   Chloride balance generally parallels that of sodium except in a hypochloremic state from losses of gastric acid.

4.   Calcium

      a.   Maintained at 4-5.5 mEq/liter (ionized calcium).

      b.   Most calcium is in bone with only the extracellular fluid amount being physiologically active.

      c.   Influences on urinary calcium excretions include parathyroid hormone, metabolic alkalosis, hypophosphatemia and metabolic acidosis, depletion of Vitamin D, absorption of small bowel calcium, etc.

C.   Acid base balance

    1.   Buffering systems in RBCs and body fluids immediately offset changes in acid-base balance.

    2.   Pulmonary ventilation promptly adjusts the excretion carbon dioxide.

    3.   Renal tubular function modulates urinary excretion or conservation of acid or base with time.

a. The Henderson-Hasselbach equation is shown below:

$$pH = pK^a + \log \frac{[HCO_3]}{[H_2CO_3]}$$

$$pH = 6.1 + \log \frac{[HCO_3]}{[0.03 \times Pco_2]}$$

III. Abnormalities

A. Fluids

1. Volume depletion

a. "Tennis score" correlates with clinical signs and symptoms of fluid loss.

(1) 0-15% loss - minimal signs and symptoms - decreased pulse pressure.

(2) 15-30% loss - tachycardia, orthostatic hypotension, moderate decrease in urine output, elevation of hematocrit.

(3) 30-40% loss - stupor or coma, eyes sunken, pulse rapid, weak and thready, hypotension, oliguria pronounced.

(4) > 40% loss - progressive coma, hypotension and death.

2. Volume excess

a. Clinical picture depends on the cause, nature and severity of the challenge and signs can range widely from simple weight gain and small decreases in hemoglobin and hematocrit to frank congestive heart failure, pulmonary edema, pleural effusion and congestive hepatomegaly.

B. Electrolytes

1. Sodium

a. Hyponatremia

(1)   Most commonly due to accumulation of excess water from hypotonic fluid replacement or retention of excess water due to enhanced ADH activity - numerous other causes.

(2)   CNS symptoms predominant including weakness, fatigue, hyperactive deep tendon reflexes, muscle twitches, etc - eventually leading to convulsions, coma and areflexia.

(3)   Most cases of dilutional hyponatremia can be treated by withholding fluids. Severe hyponatremia may need hypertonic sodium solutions.

b.   Hypernatremia

(1)   Less common than hyponatremia - most commonly the result of loss of body fluids or decreased excretion of sodium.

(2)   Symptoms associated include restlessness, weakness, decreased salivation, dry mucous membranes, dry flushed skin, decreased skin turgor, hyperpyrexia, tachycardia, hypotension and ultimately coma, convulsions and death.

(3)   Calculation of water deficit is important with replacement of hypotonic fluids - staged with no more than 1/2 in the first 8 hours, the remainder over the next 16 hours.

2.   Potassium

a.   Hypokalemia

(1)   Most commonly due to abnormal losses of potassium from gastric or intestinal content losses, enhanced aldosterone activity with associated alkalosis, diuresis with pharmacologic agents, etc.

(2)   Clinical manifestations reflect the role of potassium in muscle and nerve function. Most severe are cardiac arrhythmias with low voltage, flattening of the T-waves, prominent U-waves, prolonged P-R interval and widening of the QRS complex. Oral or intravenous potassium chloride salts may be used for replacement. Should be replaced at no more than 10-20 mEq/hour and should be on cardiac monitor at upper levels of replacement.

b. Hyperkalemia

(1) Most common cause of hyperkalemia is decreased renal excretion of potassium - excessive intake or extensive trauma with rhabdomyolysis can cause hyperkalemia, as well.

(2) The most important symptom complex relates to cardiotoxicity, manifested by peaked T-waves, diminished P-waves, increased P-R intervals, heart block, widening of the QRS complex and decreased S-T segments.

(3) Treatment of hyperkalemia involves maintenance of cell membrane function and reduction of total body potassium.

(a) Calcium gluconate and insulin/glucose/bicarb are combinations that may stabilize cardiac cell membranes and shift potassium back into the cells temporarily.

(b) Use of sodium polystyrene sulfonate (Kayexalate), a cation-exchange resin, diuretics or dialysis will all decrease total body potassium level.

3. Calcium

a. Hypocalcemia

(1) May be seen after surgically induced hypoparathyroidism or due to acute pancreatitis or inadequate absorption with inflammatory bowel disease or pancreatic exocrine dysfunction.

(2) Clinical manifestations include circumoral paresthesias, numbness and tingling of the tips of the fingers and muscle cramps (Chvostek's sign and Trousseau's sign) - EKG may show prolongation of Q-T interval.

(3) Treatment involves replacement of calcium deficit orally or intravenously and vitamin D supplements.

b. Hypercalcemia

(1) The most common causes include primary or secondary hypoparathyroidism and metastatic bone cancer, as well as numerous other causes.

(2)   Symptoms include weakness, anorexia, nausea and vomiting, headaches, musculoskeletal pain, polyuria, polydipsia and eventually coma and death.

(3)   Treatment - restrict calcium, improve hydration and increase urinary diuresis with lasix, replenish magnesium, steroids to suppress calcium release from bone, use of Mithramycin to suppress bone resorption and calcium release.

C.   Acid base balance

1.   Respiratory acidosis

     a.   Large alveolar levels of $PaCO_2$ due to inadequate ventilation.

     b.   Treatment involves improving alveolar ventilation to reduce CO_2 levels and may require the use of mechanical ventilatory support.

2.   Respiratory alkalosis

     a.   Usually the consequence of pulmonary alveolar hyperventilation, i.e. apprehension, pain, hypoxia, fever, CNS injuries or elevated ammonia levels.

     b.   Treatment aimed at the underlying problem.

3.   Metabolic acidosis

     a.   Occurs because of either loss of bicarb (diarrhea, external pancreatic fistula, etc.) or from an increase in metabolic acid load, i.e. lactic acidemia secondary to cardiogenic, septic or hypovolemic shock, ischemia of tissue beds or ketoacidosis.

     b.   Results in decreased serum concentrations. Bicarbonate determination and use of anion gap can help distinguish metabolic acidosis caused by loss of bicarb from that due to accumulation of metabolic acid load.

     (1)   Anion gap = $[Na] - [Cl] + [CO_2]$

         Normal = 10-12

       c.   Treatment is aimed at underlying disorder. Hypovolemia and sepsis must be controlled. Diabetic ketoacidosis must be treated. Other severe acid loads may be treated with hemodialysis.

    4.   Metabolic alkalosis

       a.   Associated with GI or renal losses of potassium and chloride ions, leading to hypochloremic hypokalemic metabolic alkalosis.

       b.   May be associated with increased carbon dioxide retention and hypoventilation.

       c.   The clinical problems are mostly related to hypokalemia, hypochloremia and volume contraction.

       d.   Treatment - replacement of extrarenal losses of fluid and electrolytes to correct the abnormalities.

D.   Fluid and electrolyte therapy for the surgical patient.

    1.   Preoperative evaluation of abnormalities caused by the disease process and correction of those prior to anesthetic management is imperative. This includes replacement of volume and correction of the electrolyte abnormalities.

    2.   Intraoperative therapy is directed toward maintenance of normal circulating volumes. An open peritoneum loses large amounts of insensible loss (200-300 cc's/hour) and handling of the intestine induces an isotonic fluid loss into the interstitial spaces, both requiring replacement during the intraoperative procedure.

    3.   Postoperative therapy is again directed toward maintenance of satisfactory intravascular fluid volume with normal renal output and normal electrolytes.

       a.   Mechanical ventilation greatly decreases the need for insensible water loss replacement.

       b.   Normal elevated levels of ADH and aldosterone postoperatively should limit the amount of potassium needed and the amount of fluid needed.

IV.   Nutrition

A.   Normal caloric requirements

1. Range from 30-80 K cal/kg/day depending on age and stress.

2. Harris-Benedict equations are used for resting metabolic rate.

3. Requirements can be based on 35 K cal/kg/day increased by 12% after major surgery, by 20-50% during sepsis and up to 100% with major burns.

4. Protein requirements for a normal active man are .9-1.5 grams/kg/body weight daily. Minimum of 500 ml of 10% lipid emulsion must be given twice weekly to prevent an essential fatty acid deficiency, maximum of 60% of calories can be given as lipid emulsions.

5. Fat soluble vitamins (A, D, E and K) and water soluble vitamins are important for replacement and can be given parenterally or enterally.

6. Trace elements including iron, iodine, cobalt, zinc, copper, selenium and chromium need to be replaced as well as others.

B. Sources of nutritional replacement

1. Enteral alimentation

    a. Can be infused through tubes passed through the nose, directly into the stomach or into the small intestine.

    b. Elemental diets are high osmolar, expensive solutions of synthetic aminoacids that can be infused through a small catheter directly into the small bowel. Absorption of single aminoacids in the small bowel mucosa is reasonable.

    c. Semielemental diets are low in osmolality, have good absorption in the small bowel as dipeptides and tripeptides and are less expensive than elemental diets. They do, however, need a larger tube for infusion.

    d. Modular formulas - MCT (medium chain triglycerides), etc. are particular types of formulas to replace specific deficits.

    e. The complications of enteral feedings are similar to those detailed with parenteral nutrition and include diarrhea causing hyperosmotic non-ketotic dehydration and coma, electrolyte and mineral deficiency, catheter problems with dislocation and spillage into abdominal cavity, infection and abscess formation, small bowel obstruction, etc.

2. Total parenteral nutrition (TPN)

    a. Consists of replacement of adequate volume and electrolytes and, in addition, a large amount of aminoacid solution with high levels of a non-protein source of calories, most commonly glucose.

    b. Because the fluid is very hyperosmotic, parenteral nutrition needs to be given through a high flow vein such as the subclavian or superior vena cava.

    c. Because of the high carbohydrate load and osmolality, fluid is started slowly and kept at a steady rate. It should not be interrupted during continuous infusion and when discontinuing TPN the rate must be tapered slowly over a day or two. Tapering up and down of the rate allows time for pancreatic insulin levels to adjust to the varying glucose loads.

    d. Careful monitoring of electrolytes and fluid volume is vital to prevent complications.

    e. Complications include:

        (1) Problems with placement of the catheter including pneumothorax, hemothorax, carotid injury, tracheal injury, brachial plexus injury, etc.

        (2) Infections with the line, usually Staph species.

        (3) Infection in the solution itself, especially fungal organisms (Candida).

        (4) Metabolic problems with the solutions or rate of administration, including hyperosmolar, nonketotic dehydration and coma and fluid and electrolyte abnormalities.

    f. Special types of aminoacid solutions

        (1) Branch-chain in aminoacids are used in hepatic failure patients.

        (2) Fluids replacing only essential aminoacids (to decrease the nitrogen load) are particularly useful for renal failure patients.

SHOCK

I. Introduction

A. Shock can be defined as that state in which the metabolic demands of the cells (primarily oxygen) are not met by the supply of nutrients from the body. This results in metabolic dysfunction of cellular activities and is reversible when treated aggressively in the early state but when allowed to continue results in cellular death, organ damage and death of the patient. Although commonly associated with hypotension, shock may be present without hypotension and may not necessarily be present with hypotension.

B. Pathophysiology

   1. The decrease in intravascular volume results in a decrease in mean arterial pressure and rising heart rate.

   2. Immediate result of hypovolemic episode is a surge of catecholamines from the adrenal glands, resulting in peripheral vasoconstriction and tachycardia to increase cardiac output.

   3. The juxtaglomerular apparatus of the kidney detects the decreased blood pressure, stimulating the release of renin which is converted to angiotensin causing peripheral vasoconstriction, as well as stimulating the release of aldosterone.

      a. These two actions result in elevated peripheral vascular resistance to raise the systolic blood pressure as well as increase intravascular volume, due to aldosterone effects of sodium and water retention.

4.   Increased secretion of antidiuretic hormone from the pituitary, also enhances intravascular volume by renal absorption of water.

5.   Numerous other hormones including the corticoids, growth hormone and thyroid hormone are secreted in any shock state which stimulate protective mechanisms for maintenance of blood flow to the brain and the heart.

C.   Four types of pathophysiologic mechanisms leading to cellular dysfunction and death have been described and will be detailed below. The hemodynamic parameters which aid in the diagnosis of these shock groups are summarized in the following table.

Condition	BP, mmHg	P	PCWP, mmHg	Cl, liters/min/m^2	SVR, dyn/sec/cm^{-5}	O$_2$D, mL/mm	O$_2$C, mL/mm
Normal (N)	120/70	80	5-15	2.5-3.5	1000-1500	900-1200	200-300
Hypovolemia	↓	↑	↓	↓	↑	↓	↓
CHF	↑	↑	↑	↓	↑	↓	↓
Cardiogenic shock	↓	↑	↑	↓↓	↑↑	↓↓	↓↓
Sepsis	↓	↑	↓ or N	↑	↓	↑	↑ or N
Neurogenic	↓	↑ or N	↑ or N	↑ or N	↓	↑ or N	N

BP, arterial blood pressure; P, pulse; PCWP, pulmonary capillary wedge pressure; Cl, cardiac index; SVR, systemic vascular resistance; O$_2$D, oxygen delivery; O$_2$C, oxygen consumption.

II.   Hypovolemic shock

A.   General

1.   Hypovolemic shock is the most common form of shock manifested by surgical patients and represents marked reduction in oxygen delivery, resulting from diminished cardiac output because of inadequate intravascular volume.

B.   Diagnosis

1. Common clinical states associated with hypovolemic shock should induce a high index of suspicion, such as recent trauma, fever, history of vomiting or diarrhea, intra-abdominal pain, burns, etc.

2. Blood pressure and heart rate in supine, sitting and standing positions can be indicative or helpful at indicating hypovolemia.

3. Patients tend to have decreased mental function and marked decrease in urinary output.

4. Invasive hemodynamic monitoring can also be useful to aid in proving hypovolemia (refer to the table above).

C. Treatment

1. Because patients in hypovolemic shock are hypotensive due to reduced volume, it is important to replace volume as rapidly as possible.

2. Patients who have lost blood, need blood replaced, in addition to crystalloid solutions.

3. Lactated Ringer's, normal saline or plasmalyte are good balanced electrolyte solutions that can be used to replace volume until blood is available.

   a. Typed and crossmatched blood will take approximately 1 hour to be available.

   b. Typed specific blood can be obtained within 5 to 10 minutes.

   c. O negative blood is universal donor when needed urgently.

4. Fluid resuscitation can be assessed with the invasive central lines (CVP and Swan-Ganz), as well as urinary output, mental function, blood pressure and heart rate.

5. Correction of the underlying problem may then be undertaken safely, whether it be an intra-abdominal process or injuries with blood loss.

6. Inotropic agents in patients with hypovolemic shock are very seldom of any benefit.

III. Cardiogenic shock

A. Definition

1. Cardiogenic shock is present when severe reduction in oxygen delivery is secondary to marked impairment of myocardial function.

2. The most common etiology for this is ischemic heart disease or arrhythmia.

B. Diagnosis

1. In a patient with suggestive history of an etiology of cardiogenic shock, invasive monitoring is very important in identifying the presence of cardiogenic shock.

2. See table under I.C.

3. Hemodynamic hallmarks of shock distinguishing it from hypovolemic shock are marked decrease in cardiac output and cardiac index, as well as increase in filling pressures including pulmonary artery wedge pressure and CVP.

C. Treatment

1. Treatment involves efforts to maximize myocardial performance with the least amount of myocardial oxygen consumption.

2. Concepts involved include assuring reasonable levels of pre-load, i.e., central venous pressure and intravascular volume while reducing high levels of systemic vascular resistance.

   a. Diuretics and vasodilators can be used to decrease the after load and to maintain normal filling volumes in the heart.

3. Increased contractility of the heart to improve the performance of the cardiac muscles.

   a. Three drugs commonly used for contractility are dobutamine, dopamine and isoproterenol.

4. In severe cases, mechanical intervention to improve cardiac function and reduce myocardial oxygen consumption can be helpful in the form of intra-aortic balloon pumping.

IV. Septic shock

A.   Early septic shock (warm shock)

    1.   Most commonly manifested in patients with overwhelming sepsis due to gram negative organisms but may also be seen with gram positive and fungal organisms.

    2.   In addition to hypotension and tachycardia, patients with early septic shock have marked decrease in peripheral vascular resistance because of endotoxin dismantling of peripheral neurovascular regulatory activity so that these patients are warm and pink rather than constricted and cool.

    3.   This is marked by greatly increased cardiac output that may reach 10 liters per minute.

    4.   As the shock progresses, there is decreasing compensation by the heart as the myocardium function decreases, resulting in lower cardiac output.

        a.   Ultimately vasoconstriction occurs creating cool extremities. The patient takes on more characteristics of a patient with hypovolemic shock.

B.   Treatment

    1.   Treatment is directed toward the underlying etiology, as well as the hemodynamic problems.

    2.   The underlying etiology must be treated with antibiotics and drainage of any abscesses or debridement of any necrotic materials.

    3.   Fluid resuscitation and inotropic agents to support the heart may also be important during this phase of septic shock.

IV.   **Neurogenic shock**

A.   General

    1.   Neurogenic shock is used to describe hypotension secondary to central nervous system dysfunction.

    2.   This type of shock is most commonly seen in trauma patients and may be combined with other problems such as hypovolemia, tension pneumothorax, cardiac tamponade, etc.

3.   Neurogenic shock results primarily from the disruption of the sympathetic nervous system with resultant relative hypovolemia due to widespread vasodilatation.

4.   This problem can be improved by placing the patient in the Trendelenburg's position, using intravascular volume replacement, or giving some sympathomimetic agents to improve peripheral and vasoconstriction.

CLOTTING DISORDERS AND USE OF BLOOD PRODUCTS

I.   Clotting disorders

    A.   Screening

        1.   History of previous bleeding problems is the most helpful screening test in evaluating patients with possible bleeding problems.

        2.   Other screening tests that are commonly helpful in patients without a history of bleeding disorder after surgical procedures include a platelet count, prothrombin time (PT) and partial prothrombin time (PTT).

        3.   Numerous other tests for evaluation of hemostasis can be undertaken, depending upon the abnormality of these and the history.

                a.   Bleeding time - actual prolonged bleeding time is often associated with platelet aggregation disorder.

                b.   Thrombin time - evaluates fibrinogen to fibrin conversion with an external source of thrombin. Used to evaluate DIC and chronic liver disease.

                c.   Specific evaluations of clotting factors may be undertaken to identify specific deficiencies such as Type A hemophilia and von Willebrand's disease, etc.

        4.   Acquired bleeding disorders are most commonly associated with use of medications.

a.   Aspirin and non-steroidal anti-inflammatory medications commonly interfere with platelet function.

b.   Exogenous heparin is used for anticoagulation and causes prolongation of the PTT.

c.   Coumadin causes decreased synthesis of liver-manufactured clotting factors (II, VII, IX and X) - causes prolongation of the PT (and PTT to a lesser extent).

d.   Any chronic liver disease interferes with liver function and may cause prolonged PT and bleeding abnormalities.

e.   Acquired thrombocytopenia may be due to decreased platelet production due to bone marrow failure, increased destruction of platelets by increased activity by the spleen, splenic pooling of platelets and an enlarged abnormal spleen or any combination of these disorders, such as alcoholic liver failure.

Coagulation Pathways

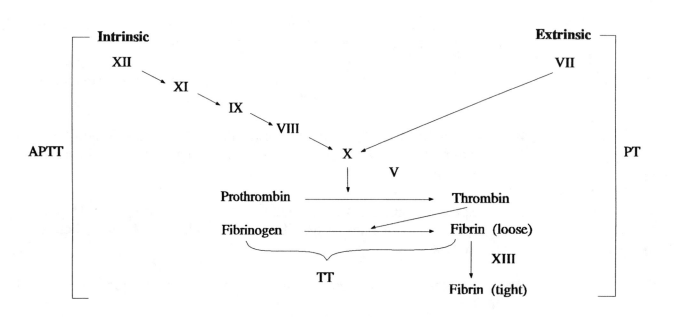

B.   Causes of surgical bleeding

1.   Pre-existing hemostatic defects as detailed above or acquired bleeding disorder may be a cause of intraoperative bleeding problems.

2.   Shock and extensive trauma may be associated with disseminated intravascular coagulation and result in oozing capillaries and massive blood loss.

3.   Rapid transfusion of 10 units or more of stored blood over 4 to 6 hours may result in abnormal bleeding because of reduced numbers of platelets, decreased coagulation factors and hypothermia.

4.   50% of postoperative bleeding is due to inadequate hemostasis during surgery. Other causes of bleeding during surgery include circulating heparin remaining after bypass procedures, shock resulting in DIC and factor deficiencies.

5.   Secondary fibrinolysis may be the cause of abnormal bleeding due to disseminated intravascular coagulation. This is often activated by shock, sepsis, allergic reactions, etc.

    a.   The diagnosis of DIC is established by detecting diminished levels of coagulation factors, platelets and presence of fibrin split products.

II.   Blood replacement therapy

A.   Packed red blood cells

1.   When patients have lost red cell volume, the usual replacement is with packed red blood cells, which have a volume of approximately 250 cc's and hematocrit of approximately 70%.

2.   Blood group and type must be taken into consideration when red cells are given, including ABO blood groups and RH factors.

    a.   Universal donor red cells are O negative red blood cells when type specific or typed and crossmatched blood cannot be made available.

3.   Tests for transmission of infectious agents including hepatitis virus, HIV and CMV virus are done routinely so that the risk is extremely small.

    a.   Risk for transmission of disease increases as the number of transfused units increases.

B.   Fresh frozen plasma

    1.   Fresh frozen plasma is used when replacement of coagulation factors is important.

    2.   Can be used to reverse the effects of Coumadin as it rapidly replaces II, VII, IX and X.

    3.   Fresh frozen plasma can be used in a non specific manner, not requiring cross matching. Risk of transmission of disease is similar with red blood cells.

C.   Cryoprecipitate

    1.   Measures 5 to 30 ml in a single plastic bag and is rich in factor VIII, fibrinogen and fibronectin.

    2.   Concentrated from pooled sources of plasma and therefore has a slightly increased risk of transmission of disease.

    3.   Is particularly useful in the treatment hemophilia A and von Willebrand's disease.

D.   Factor VIII concentrates

    1.   Useful for treating hemophilia A but not in the treatment of von Willebrand's disease.

    2.   Because of additional concentration from various sources of plasma, the risk of hepatitis virus is increased.

E.   Complications of transfusions

    1.   Immunologic transfusion reactions include:

        a.   hemolytic transfusion reaction

        b.   febrile transfusion reactions

        c.   post transfusion thrombocytopenia

        d.   antiphylactic shock

        e.   urticaria

f.   graft versus host disease

2.   Symptoms of immediate hemolytic reaction include fever, constrictive sensation of the chest, pain in the lumbar region and fever, hypotension, hemoglobinuria, bleeding due to DIC and renal failure.

3.   Transfusion should be stopped immediately, documentation of clinical information double checked, blood samples taken from the patient to re-check typing and for free plasma hemoglobin.

    a.   Cultures of the patient's blood and investigation for DIC are important.

    b.   Management of hypotension with volume expanders such as lactated Ringer's and vasoactive drugs and good renal function maintained with a diuretic therapy.

SURGICAL INFECTIONS

I. Classification of surgical wounds

Wound	Bacterial Contaminants	Source of Contamination	Infection Frequency	Examples
Clean	Gram positive	OR environment, surgical team, patient's skin	3%	Inguinal hernia, thyroidectomy, mastectomy
Clean-contaminated	Polymicrobial	Endogenous colonization of the patient	5-15%	Common duct exploration, elective colon resection, gastrectomy for carcinoma
Contaminated	Polymicrobial	Gross contamination	15-40%	"Spill" during elective GI surgery, perforated gastric ulcer
Dirty	Polymicrobial	Established infection	40%	Drainage of intraabdominal abscess, resection of infarcted intestine.

II. Pathogenesis of infection

A. Anything that leads to increased bacterial virulence (numerous adjuvants fall into this category) or anything that reduces host defense may lead to increased chances of infection.

B. Numerous adjuvants of bacterial virulence include presence of hemoglobin, dead tissue, foreign body, decreased oxygen concentration in the tissues, etc.

C. Systemic factors such as shock, hypovolemia and hypoxia deter a host defense as well as the coexistence of systemic problems such as diabetes, obesity, starvation, alcoholic liver disease, systemic drug therapy with corticosteroids or cancer chemotherapy, etc.

III. Prevention of surgical infection

A. Most surgical infections stem directly from the patients' own endogenous microflora and depend on the degree of contamination present at the time of the procedure.

B. Personnel in the operating room are the most common source of bacterial contamination in this setting. Thus, the use of masks, gowns, gloves, operating room air filtering system, etc. are employed.

C. Prophylactic antibiotics are used for clean contaminated and contaminated wounds.

   1. Should be started at least 1 to 2 hours prior to the operating time to allow for adequate tissue concentration.

   2. Prophylactic antibiotics are carried through the operation and for no more than 24 hours postoperatively.

   3. Shaving prior to the operating room should not be undertaken.

   4. Elective colon surgery should be done with mechanical bowel prep as well as either systemic antibiotics or orally administered, poorly absorbed antibiotics to reduce enteric bacteria within the colon.

D. When dealing with contaminated wounds and dirty procedures, risk of wound infections exceeds 15 to 20% and therapeutic antibiotics are then used beginning preoperatively and extending until the infection is well contained. Additionally, the wound surface is left open after closing the fascia so that the wound can be managed with wet to dry dressings.

IV. Community acquired infections

A. Skin - skin structure infections.

   1. Soft tissue infections following minor cuts or abrasions may present with spreading cellulitis, usually represent infection in the group of Streptococci or Staphylococci.

   2. These wounds may be more severe and involve necrotizing streptococcal gangrene or widespread cellulitis and lymphangitis, necessitating increased doses of antibiotics toward these bacteria.

B. Peri-rectal abscess

1.   A commonly encountered cutaneous infection of the perirectal tissues (obstructed perianal glands) containing mixed enteric flora bacteria. Wide spectrum antibiotics are used after incision and drainage of the abscess.

C.   Biliary tract infections

    1.   Usually the result of obstruction of the cystic or occasionally, common bile duct.

    2.   Involved bacteria include Escherichia coli, Klebsiella species, enterococci and Clostridia.

    3.   Cephalosporins are particularly highly concentrated in bile and are very useful for these infections as are other antibiotics for these organisms.

D.   Acute peritonitis

    1.   Usually the result of mechanical perforation of the hollow viscus, representing a mixed flora infection of the peritoneal cavity. Anaerobes and gram negative enteric bacteria are the most common and antibiotics directed toward these should be initiated.

E.   Other community acquired infections

    1.   Breast abscess - most common in lactating mothers. Characterized by local pain, swelling and redness and most often caused by staphylococcal infections.

    2.   Gas gangrene - Clostridium perfringens infection of the soft tissues may include cellulitis and myonecrosis, marked by a brown, watery drainage from the wound site and marked tenderness around the wound. Very severe infection requiring wide debridement and antibiotic dosage.

    3.   Tetanus - unusual infection caused by the exotoxin of <u>Clostridium tetani</u>. Management includes debridement of devitalized contaminated tissue along with immunization and penicillin.

    4.   Hand infections - result from trauma (especially bites) and mixed flora invasions. Penicillin treatment and wide drainage are indicated.

IV.   **Hospital acquired infection**

    A.   Pulmonary infection

1. Postoperative atelectasis leading to fever from entrapped bacteria are very common in the first 48 hours after a general anesthetic.

    a. Respiratory therapy by the nurses, family members or respiratory technicians to induce deep breathing, coughing, etc., will resolve this.

2. Postoperative pneumonitis may be ventilator associated, particularly in critically ill patients. Most common organism is gram negative species, especially Pseudomonas and Serratia.

    a. Mechanical cleansing of the bronchial tree and high dose antibiotics, along with overall nutritional status are important in patient salvage of these very serious infections.

3. Aspiration is an ever present risk in the postoperative patient.

    a. Aspiration leads to chemical damage of the lung and introduction of local bacteria and can be best prevented by liberal use of NG decompression of GI tract.

B. Urinary tract infection

1. Patients with indwelling Foley catheters will often develop bladder and urethral infections particularly with gram negative organisms (E. coli).

2. Most positive cultures will clear after removal of the catheter but also require systemic antibiotics.

C. Wound infection

1. The wound is always a consideration, particularly after third to fifth day, as a source of fever.

2. Signs and symptoms include tenderness, redness, heat, swelling around the wound, discharge of pus from the wound is definitive.

3. Required treatment required includes opening the wound, evacuation of pus and debridement along with systemic antibiotics.

D. Intra-abdominal infection

1. Abscess formation may occur after intra-abdominal operations, depending on the type of operation performed.

2. These become manifest at five to seven days with spiking fevers, associated systemic illness (tachycardia, diaphoresis, anorexia, weakness, etc).

3. X-rays of the abdomen and CT scans are helpful in identifying intra-abdominal abscess, as are Gallium-67 scans.

4. Abdominal exploration of postoperative abdominal patient with abdominal tenderness and fever, is often the only way to definitively diagnose the problem.

5. Abscesses identified on CT scan may occasionally be drained with percutaneous placement of catheters and irrigation of the cavity.

E. Intravascular device associated bacteremia

1. Bacteremia may be associated with any invasive intravascular catheters and devices.

2. Clearing bacteria from these devices is very difficult as the intravascular antibiotics pass by very quickly and it is very difficult for leukocytes to deal with the bacteria harbored on these devices.

3. Fevers which have no other source and cannot be eliminated with antibiotics usually require removal of these indwelling devices to clear the infection.

4. Staphyloccal aureus or epidermidis are the most common types of organisms involved in these infections.

MULTIPLE TRAUMA

I.   Primary survey - ABCDE

    A.   Airway

         1.   Chin lift jaw thrust

         2.   Oral airway

         3.   Nasal airway

         4.   Orotracheal/nasotracheal intubation

         5.   Cricothyrotomy

    B.   Breathing

         1.   Evaluate for hemothorax, pneumothorax or tension pneumothorax.

         2.   Life threatening problems of breathing

               a.   Tension pneumothorax - hypoxia associated with decreased breath sounds on the side of the tension pneumothorax with deviation of the trachea away from the side of the tension pneumothorax, resulting in rapid cardiovascular collapse. Treatment includes large gauge needle inserted into the second intercostal space anteriorly to relieve the pressure, followed by a chest tube.

               b.   Simple pneumothorax - decreased breath sounds on side of injury with resulting hypoxia and hyperresonance on the opposite side, no tracheal deviation, treatment with chest tube.

      c.   Massive hemothorax - results from injury to any vessel either in the chest wall or mediastinum, associated with hypoxia, decreased breath sounds and hyporesonance on percussion of the involved side. Treatment involves placement of chest tube and rapid fluid resuscitation.

      d.   Flail chest - associated with multiple broken ribs, often broken in two positions so that during inspiration the chest wall caves in and during expiration the chest wall flaps out, results in hypoxia and agitation. Treated with chest tube and positive ventilation when necessary.

      e.   Cardiac tamponade - associated with anterior chest trauma, resulting in elevated jugular distention (elevated CVP), decreased blood pressure and decreased heart sounds (Beck's triad). Water bottle heart on chest x-ray. Treated with aspiration of blood from the pericardial space, usually only a small amount needs to be removed (50 cc's).

C.   Circulation

      1.   Start two large bore (14-16 gauge) peripheral IV's with lactated Ringer's or normal saline.

      2.   Adequacy of volume resuscitation gauged by mental function, blood pressure and heart rate, urinary output, central venous pressure or pulmonary artery wedge pressure.

D.   Disability

      1.   Careful neurologic evaluation for acute neurologic deterioration.

E.   Exposure

      1.   Remove all of the patients clothing; be sure to log roll the patient to examine his back.

II.   **Secondary survey**

      A.   General

      1.   After the initial primary survey and immediate correction of any problems identified during the primary survey, begin a careful review of the patient's history and physical exam from head to toe, front and back. Most neurologic,

chest, abdominal and extremity injuries are identified and cared for during the secondary survey.

2. Frequent repeated reassessments of the patient's airway, breathing, circulation and neurologic status are important during the secondary survey. Any deterioration should prompt return to the primary survey and treatment of those major life-threatening injuries.

B. Head and spine injury

1. Closed head injury may result in space-occupying lesions such as intracerebral hematoma, subdural hematoma or epidural hematoma.

   a. All are marked by focal neurologic deficit and all have the risk of tentorial herniation if further brain edema occurs.

   b. All use CT scanning or MRI scanning for diagnosis.

   c. All may be treated by surgical intervention to relieve the underlying pressure.

2. Diffuse cerebral contusion is the most common closed injury resulting in diffuse non-focal CNS deficit. Recovery is variable and largely dependent upon intracerebral pressure and edema. Is generally not helped by surgical intervention but may receive some benefit with mannitol or decadron to decrease swelling in the normal brain.

3. Glasgow coma scale is used to predict neurologic recovery. It includes the major categories of eye opening, verbal response and best motor response with better prognoses in patients with higher levels of spontaneity, orientation and following of commands.

4. Any patient with severe head trauma should be suspected of having cervical spine trauma.

   a. Requires good lateral C-spine revealing all seven cervical vertebral bodies.

   b. Patient must have had his C-spine held rigid until instability of the cervical spine can be ruled out.

   c. Any suspected injury to the spinal cord resulting in distal paralysis or unstable vertebral injuries must be treated with immobilization and

    c.   Any suspected injury to the spinal cord resulting in distal paralysis or unstable vertebral injuries must be treated with immobilization and relative dehydration to help reduce swelling until definitive repair can be undertaken.

    5.   Spinal fluid leaks may be detected with otorrhea or rhinorrhea. Periorbital ecchymoses (raccoon eyes) and paramastoid ecchymosis (Battle's sign) and hemotympanum; are all indicative of basilar skull fractures.

C.   Thoracic injuries

    1.   Tension pneumothorax, simple pneumothorax, hemothorax, flail chest and cardiac tamponade are all reviewed in I.B. above.

    2.   Penetrating trauma to the thorax most often results in simple pneumothorax or hemopneumothorax and generally only requires treatment with chest tube.

    3.   Injury to the great vessels in the thorax often results in death very quickly. In patients who make it to the hospital, this injury usually requires aortography for definitive diagnosis and treatment.

    4.   In patients who arrive in the emergency room alive, trauma to the great vessels usually does not cause significant hypotension problems.

    5.   Pulmonary contusion often becomes manifest 1 to 4 hours post injury resulting in hypoxemia and worsening of the chest x-ray and is treated by careful judicious use of fluids guided by central pressure monitoring and treatment of any potential infections.

    6.   Myocardial contusion, particularly with anterior chest trauma, is marked by S-T elevations and elevated CPK fractions, suggesting myocardial infarction.

        a.   Right ventricle most commonly involved. Arrhythmias may occur.

        b.   Requires monitoring in an ICU for 42 to 78 hours to identify and treat arrhythmias.

    7.   Radiographic signs suggesting thoracic aortic injuries include a widened mediastinum, loss of aortic knob, pleural cap, deviation of trachea to the right, fracture of the first or second rib or scapula, elevation of right mainstem bronchus, depression of left mainstem bronchus, obliteration of aortopulmonary window, deviation of the esophagus to the left.

8. Esophageal injuries - esophageal ruptures can be identified by esophagograms or esophagoscopy. They may be suspected by mediastinal crunch (Hamman's sign) and fever. Particulate matter may be found in a left pleural effusion which develops.

    a. These injuries if not treated early are frequently fatal.

    b. Surgical repair with wide drainage and occasionally deviation of GI tract is indicated.

9. Traumatic diaphragmatic hernia may occur after blunt or penetrating trauma, resulting in tears in the diaphragm which may allow intra-abdominal contents into the chest.

    a. More common on the left than on the right.

    b. Results in respiratory distress, requires repair usually through an intra-abdominal approach.

D. Abdominal injuries

1. The abdominal cavity may extend from the nipple line (with elevated diaphragm) all the way down to the bottom of the pelvis.

2. Evidence of intra-abdominal injury on examination with either significant abdominal pain or abdominal distention with hypotension should be indication for immediate laparotomy.

3. In the unconscious patient with a benign abdominal exam, the patient who is about to be removed from your ability to frequently examine the patient, i.e., going to the OR for repair of extremity injury; or the patient on whom the exam is questionable might be served by having peritoneal lavage.

    a. Peritoneal lavage is usually performed using an open technique below the umbilicus, instilling 1,000 cc's of lactated Ringer's into the abdominal cavity and allowing it to return. The presence of gross blood or intestinal contents on aspiration is indicative of a positive exam.

    b. Also indicative of positive exam is 10^5 red cells, 500 white blood cells, amylase greater than serum amylase, bilirubin greater than serum bilirubin.

      c.   A negative peritoneal lavage does not rule out injuries to retroperitoneal organs, such as pancreas, duodenum, aorta, vena cava or kidneys.

4. A CT scan of the abdominal cavity can also be very good for identifying intra-abdominal injuries.

5. Blunt trauma with hemorrhage most commonly results from injury to the spleen or liver.

      a.   Massive splenic injuries disrupting the body of the spleen and particularly the hilum should be treated with splenectomy. Lesser degrees of injury may be repaired.

      b.   Liver lacerations (most commonly) can be treated with suture control of the bleeding sites and/or packing of the wounds. Massive liver injuries may require lobectomy.

6. Other blunt injuries in the abdomen include rupture of the small bowel (associated with seat belt injuries) and destruction of any of the major vessels and rupture of the kidneys.

7. Penetrating abdominal trauma occurs with gunshot wounds, knife wounds or other sharp instruments.

      a.   All gunshot wounds to the abdomen require laparotomy because of the danger of blast effect injuring organs not directly in the path of the missile.

      b.   Stab wounds that result in diffuse pain, significant bleeding or extrusion of intra-abdominal contents require laparotomy (some centers would use peritoneal lavage in patients with lesser degrees of injury to identify those which require laparotomy).

E. Extremity injuries

1. Assessment of distal pulses and neurologic function is most important in any extremity injury.

2. Stabilization of fractures or dislocation of extremities is important, particularly after alignment of those fractures that have been displaced.

3.   Femoral fractures and pelvic fractures may be associated with hemorrhagic shock without overt external signs of the massive blood loss that can occur in these areas.

4.   Orthopedic injuries particularly prone to be associated with neurovascular injuries are supracondylar fractures of the humerus and femur and dislocation of the knee.

F.   Tetanus prophylaxis

If the patient's immunization history is unknown or patient has been immunized more than ten years previously, should receive 0.5 cc's of absorbed toxoid with most non-tetanus prone wounds. Those with very significant tetanus prone wounds should also receive 250 units of tetanus immune globulin. Patients who have been immunized more than 5 years previously and have tetanus prone wounds should also receive 0.5 cc's of absorbed toxoid. No therapy is needed in patients, who have been fully immunized with the last booster within ten years (who have a non-tetanus prone wound).

BURNS

I. Types and classification of burn injuries

A. Types of burn injuries

1. Scalds

2. Flame burn

3. Radiation burn

4. Electrical burn

B. Classification of depths of burn injury

1. First degree - involves burn of superficial layers of skin, is painful, does not result in blisters or scarring, example - sunburn.

2. Second degree - more severe injury of the dermis and epidermis resulting in a red, painful wound which blisters and weeps.

3. Third degree - burn involving deeper layers of tissue with total destruction of dermal, subdermal elements including nerves, resulting in a white, dry, hard, painless wound. These injuries will not heal by themselves and require significant contraction or skin grafts to heal.

4. Fourth degree - severe burn involving all layers of the dermal and subcutaneous tissue down to and including bone and tendon, requires major reconstructive procedures to repair.

5. Electrical burn - may be associated with any depth of wound.

a. Entry site, exit site may be the only external manifestations of the injury, however severe muscle injury may occur subcutaneously that requires fluid resuscitation and careful electrolyte balance.

6. Inhalation injury is manifested by singed nasal hairs, carbonaceous sputum, hypoxia, tachypnea and other history suggesting possible inhalation injury, including flame burn in a closed environment, explosion, etc.

a. May need to be managed with endotracheal intubation and mechanical ventilation.

II. Treatment

A. Fluid resuscitation

1. Rule of 9's

a. The upper extremities and the head and neck each make up 9% of total body surface area, while the anterior and posterior torso and the lower extremities each make up 18%; genitalia make up 1%. This applies for adults and must be modified for infants.

2. Parkland formula for fluid resuscitation - 4 cc's/kg/% burned in addition to normal maintenance fluids given totally as crystalloid with 1/2 the volume given in the first 8 hours post burn and the second 1/2 given over the next 16 hours.

a. Adequacy of fluid resuscitation is judged by urinary output, central venous pressure monitoring, blood gases, mental function and serum electrolytes.

b. Colloid replacement begins in the second 24 hours depending on the patient's hematocrit, serum albumin, etc.

3. Other fluid resuscitation recommendations are available, i.e., Brooke formula, etc.

4. Most common cause of death in the first 24 hours is inadequacy of fluid resuscitation.

B. Wound care

1.   Initial management involves removal of dead or necrotic tissue. Coverage of the wound with topical antibiotic agents (Silvadene, etc.).

2.   Hydrotherapy used commonly to help with debridement and cleaning of the wound.

3.   Early skin grafting with split thickness skin grafts can be helpful.

4.   Firm eschars involving thorax or extremities may lead to compartment syndromes or respiratory difficulties requiring escharotomies.

5.   Antibiotics reserved for use after skin grafting or in the presence of systemic infection with wound biopsies having greater than 10^5 organisms present.

6.   Most common cause of death after the initial resuscitative phase is sepsis.

C.   General measures

1.   In addition to the above wound care, fluid resuscitation is important to maintain adequate nutrition in severely burned patients whose catabolic needs may exceed 5 to 6 thousand calories per day.

2.   Extensive rehabilitation with physical therapy, occupational therapy, etc. may be needed to help wound contractures and to rehabilitate the patient.

WOUND HEALING

I.   Pathophysiology

   A.   Normal healing

   1.   Inflammatory phase (also substrate phase, lag phase, exudative phase)

   a.   Consists of aggregation of platelets, polymorphonuclearcytes and macrophages to occlude damaged blood vessels and begin phagocytosis of foreign bodies. Release of local vasoactive hormones such as bradykinin, along with activation of the complement pathway, induces white cell migration and induction of macrophage activity. This local hormonal milieu includes angiogenesis growth hormone to stimulate the development of new blood vessels and macrophage derived growth factor which stimulates replication of fibroblasts. In 1° wound healing, this lasts approximately 4 days.

   2.   Proliferative phase

   a.   Proliferation of fibroblasts with extensive collagen production and proliferation of angiogenesis with extensive capillary production are the main thrust of this phase. Macrophages have destroyed most of the invasive bacteria and other foreign bodies in the wound and the wound now becomes stabilized and rich in vasculature. This is the so-called granulation tissue.

   b.   Proliferative phase extends from the end of the inflammatory stage (48-72 hours) and extends until full epithelization occurs.

    c.   Epithelization also occurs during this phase, depending on the size of the denuded wound. Epithelial cells migrate approximately 1 mm per day toward the center of the wound.

3.   Maturation phase

    a.   Epithelization of the wound from day 5-7 out to day 40-45, there is extensive re-working of the collagen network within the wound, aligning collagen fibrils produced by the fibroblasts in directions of skin tension, thus improving wound strength.

    b.   The maturation of the scar occurs over the next 9-12 months; resulting in flattening of the scar with the skin becoming more pale and supple.

B.   Abnormal healing

1.   Numerous factors play a role in normal and abnormal wound healing. Listed below are the items of particular importance.

Tissue oxygen supply
Presence of foreign bodies or necrotic tissue
Widely separated tissue edges
Poor macrophage function (inhibits inflammatory phase)
Diabetes mellitus
Cushing's syndrome
Glucocorticoid steroid administration
Poor nutritional support
Vitamin C deficiency (collagen bonding deficiency)
Zinc deficiency
Other vitamin and mineral deficiencies
Overwhelming sepsis
Cancer cachexia
Protein malnutrition

2.   Keloids - abnormal proliferative response to wound healing, which seems to be genetically determined seen more commonly in Blacks than Caucasians.

3.   Contracture - abnormal condition involving foreshortening of normal tissues versus contraction, which is a normal part of the inflammatory and proliferative phase of wound healing, which reduces the size of the wound.

II. Classification of wounds

A. Types of wounds

1. Laceration - clean cut edges of epidermis, dermis and varying levels of subcutaneous tissues.

2. Crush injuries which may or may not involve lacerations but involve crushing injuries to the subcutaneous tissues.

3. Abrasions - generally involves injury to the epidermis and varying levels of dermis of the skin, particularly secondary to scrape type injuries.

4. Stellate - often involve crush injury with laceration to the skin in several radial patterns, usually indicative of severe force of trauma.

B. Infection risks

1. Clean wounds - elective procedures on non-contaminated areas after adequate skin prep with sterile instruments. There is very low incidence of wound infection with these wounds (3%), example would include surgical repair of a hernia.

2. Clean contaminated wounds - involves the operation on potentially contaminated structures which have been cleaned ahead of time and would include intra-abdominal operations which do not enter the viscera. Risk of wound infection is low 5 - 15 percent.

3. Contaminated wounds - this category of wounds involves those that do enter the abdominal viscera, particularly the colon and esophagus. Risk of perioperative wound infection is moderately high (15-40 percent).

4. Gross contaminated wounds - include wounds that have been opened for a prolonged period of time, wounds involving spillage of significant intra-abdominal contents or wounds involving abscess cavities. Risk of wound infection is very high (40%).

III. Use of prophylactic antibiotics

A. Principles of use

1. Prophylactic antibiotics are administered to reduce the incidence of perioperative wound infections.

2. They must be started at least an hour prior to the incision to allow for adequate tissue concentration.

3. The antibiotic should not be continued more than 24 hours postoperatively when used in a prophylactic sense.

4. Antibiotic of choice should be that of the most commonly encountered organisms for the operation involved.

5. Prophylactic antibiotics should be used when there is a significant chance of perioperative wound infection, particularly the contaminated group of wounds and some clean contaminated operations.

6. Prophylactic antibiotics are also indicated when the consequences of infection are extremely devastating, even though the risk of infection is low. Examples: placement of prosthetic, vascular, orthopedic or cardiac materials.

IV. Wound care

A. Types of closure

1. Closure by 1° intention - indicates the wound is closed either with sutures, steri-strips or other mechanical devices after adequate irrigation and debridement.

2. 2° intention - indicates wounds that are allowed to heal while the skin edges are left open. This allows foreign materials on infected tissues to be debrided over time and prevents the chances of spreading underlying wound infections.

3. Delayed 1° closure - in which a wound is loosely closed with a few stitches and packed with gauze and left for 3 to 5 days, at which time if no pus is identified, the wound can be fully closed.

a. Delayed primary closure is used in potentially contaminated wounds in which full primary closure is not felt to be indicated, but healing by secondary intention may not be necessary.

4. Skin grafts

a. STSG - thin skin grafts used to cover large areas of absent epithelium and dermis (i.e. large burn wounds or abrasions). These grafts tend to contract and their color tends to remain abnormal compared to the surrounding tissues. In addition, thickness tends to be less than the surrounding tissues.

    b.   FTSG - used for cosmetically sensitive areas to fill in dermal defects of no greater than 1 to 2 cm in diameter because of the difficulty with blood supply. These grafts contract less, have better coloration with the surrounding tissue and blend in better.

5.   Flaps

    a.   Local pedicle flap - a segment of skin and subcutaneous tissue is locally rotated to cover the defect.

    b.   Muscle flap - the blood supply to a muscle is used and maintained to allow filling of a large tissue defect. These are usually covered with split thickness skin grafts.

    c.   Free flap: Muscle or other soft tissues are removed from one area of the body and the vascular supply is sewn in elsewhere to fill in a large soft tissue defect. Again, these are often covered with split thickness skin grafts.

B.   Wound infections

1.   Clinical manifestations usually involve erythematous, warm, painful areas surrounding the wound edges. Leakage of serosanguinous fluid from the wound edges is an early sign suggesting wound infection.

2.   Care usually involves re-opening the wound to allow drainage of the infected material.

3.   Abdominal wounds with fluid draining through the wound suggests infection of the fascia, requiring return of the patient to the operating room for irrigation, debridement and reclosure to prevent dehiscence of wound and evisceration of intestinal contents.

4.   Systemic antibiotics are often added to control surrounding cellulitis or lymphangitis.

5.   Cultures of the wound should be undertaken to determine the specific etiology to enhance adequate antibiotic coverage. Staphylococcal aureus and streptococcal species are the most common types of wound infections.

ACUTE ABDOMINAL PAIN

I. **General aspects**

   A.   Acute onset of pain in the abdomen that lasts more than six hours without other preceding events is commonly associated with some sort of surgically correctable disorder. Associated symptoms include nausea, vomiting, anorexia and fever.

   B.   The history and physical exam are the most important criteria for establishing the diagnosis. With careful evaluation of these aspects of patient interaction, a fairly limited differential diagnosis can be established which directs the pertinent laboratory and x-ray examinations.

   C.   The sequence of signs and symptoms and the age and sex of the patient are most helpful in identifying a differential diagnosis.

   D.   A careful examination not only of the abdomen, but one which also includes full evaluation of the chest and pelvis is very important for establishing the diagnosis.

II. **Acute appendicitis**

   A.   Most common in second and third decade patients.

   B.   Classic presentation begins with periumbilical diffuse abdominal pain, which in subsequent hours shifts to the right lower quadrant (McBurney's point) and becomes much more sharp and more easily localized.

   C.   Physical exam reveals right lower quadrant tenderness with rebound (psoas sign, obturator sign, Rovsing's sign) and a mild low grade fever.

   D.   Pertinent lab values include mildly elevated white blood cell count with a left shift, normal electrolytes, amylase, urinalysis, usually normal abdominal x-ray (occasional sentinel loop or fecalith).

E.   Treatment consists of appendectomy. Expect normal appendix in 15-20% of patients.

F.   In patients with normal appendices at the time of exploration look for evidence of Crohn's disease, Meckel's diverticulitis, cholecystitis, perforated ulcer, diverticulitis, ovarian or fallopian tube diseases.

III.   Pelvic inflammatory disease

A.   Occurs primarily in young, sexually active females and is due to gonorrhea, late cases may be due to enteric organisms.

B.   History commonly includes onset of bilateral lower abdominal pain within a week after menstrual periods, mild associated nausea and vomiting, commonly has associated high fever.

C.   Exam most notable for diffuse lower abdominal tenderness with poor localization. Occasional localized pain and mass with tubo-ovarian abscess. Pelvic exam reveals marked tenderness on cervical motion (chandelier sign).

D.   Laboratory notable for markedly elevated white blood cell count (15 to 20,000 with left shift), urinalysis, electrolytes, amylase, pregnancy test and abdominal x-rays usually unremarkable.

E.   Usually can be treated with antibiotics, occasionally requires removal of tubal ovarian abscess.

IV.   Ectopic pregnancy

A.   Manifest in child-bearing age females with lower abdominal pain and occasional cardiovascular collapse. Pregnancy test may or may not be positive as these may occur within two to four weeks of the last menstrual period. History of IUD, PID or previous tubal pregnancy is helpful.

B.   Presence of blood in the cul de sac is suggestive. Lower abdominal ultrasound may be helpful in the diagnosis. Classically, vaginal bleeding precedes the abdominal pain.

C.   Treatment consists of exploration and removal of the ectopic pregnancy and tube.

V.   Biliary disease

A.   Acute cholecystitis

    1.   Typical patient is middle-aged female who presents with repeated episodes of fatty food intolerance associated with right upper quadrant pain, occasional nausea and vomiting as well as mild fever.

    2.   Exam reveals tenderness in the right upper quadrant with decreased bowel sounds, mild fever and an occasional tender mass (Murphy's sign). Not usually associated with jaundice.

    3.   Laboratory usually has elevated WBCs with left shift, elevated alkaline phosphatase, occasionally mild elevation of the SGOT, LDH and bilirubin but minimal compared to the alkaline phosphatase.

    4.   Abdominal ultrasound most commonly used for diagnosis. CT scan is not usually as accurate.

    5.   Initial treatment usually includes NG suction, IV fluids, antibiotics toward the gram negative organisms that are associated with infection in the gallbladder (E. coli, Klebsiella, Serratia, Clostridium) and analgesics.

    6.   Early cholecystectomy is usually indicated with either laparoscopy or open laparotomy.

B.   Ascending cholangitis

    1.   Marked by Whipple's triad of right upper quadrant pain, fever and jaundice.

    2.   Caused by stone occluding the common bile duct.

    3.   Represents medical emergency as overwhelming sepsis can cause death of the patient within 12 to 24 hours.

    4.   Treatment consists of NG suction, IV fluids, high dose antibiotics and early decompression of the biliary tract through percutaneous drainage or operation as indicated if the patient does not improve within a few hours.

VI.   Acute pancreatitis

A.   Most commonly associated with alcohol abuse or with passage of a gallstone through the cystic duct and ampulla into the GI tract.

B.   Presents with sudden onset of acute epigastric abdominal pain radiating into the back, may be associated with acute cardiovascular collapse, fever, nausea and vomiting; often occurs soon after a meal.

C. Abdominal exam is usually indicative of upper abdominal pain that may be poorly localized. Minimal bowel sounds and usually no masses.

D. Pertinent lab includes elevated white count with left shift, hemo concentration on the electrolytes and markedly elevated serum amylase and lipase. Abdominal x-rays may show a sentinel loop or may show calcifications in the pancreas in the patient with chronic pancreatitis with recurrent episodes.

E. Initial treatment involves GI tract; rest usually involves NG suction, IV fluids, analgesics and decreased pancreatic secretion by giving secretin exogenously. Nutritional support also important.

F. Operative intervention usually indicated for complications in acute pancreatitis including development of acute pseudocyst, development of pancreatic ascites, development of pancreatic necrosis (hemorrhagic pancreatitis) or involvement of hemorrhage, etc.

VII. **Perforated duodenal ulcer**

A. Most often occurs in population groups that commonly have duodenal ulcers, however, may be the first manifestation of ulcer disease.

B. Classic onset is that of very sudden onset of excruciating abdominal pain. The patient can often pinpoint the exact time of onset. The patient may or may not have previous history of ulcer disease.

C. Examination marked by the presence of a "boardlike" abdomen which is very tense and tight with no bowel sounds.

D. Laboratory reveals elevated white cell count with left shift and a hemo concentration on the hemogram and electrolytes. Amylase may be mildly elevated. The best x-ray for demonstration of free air is upright chest x-ray. An alternative would be a left lateral decubitus abdominal x-ray. 20% of the time, no free abdominal air is demonstrated.

E. Treatment consists of NG suction, IV fluids, IV antibiotics and operative exploration to close the perforation. In patients with chronic ulcer disease, a definitive ulcer operation is usually undertaken at the same time.

VIII. **Acute diverticulitis**

A. Similar to acute appendicitis, except occurring in older age groups and more commonly associated with left lower quadrant abdominal pain.

B. History is generally that of onset of pain in the left lower quadrant with continued worsening, may be associated with fever, nausea, vomiting and occasional diarrhea or constipation complaints. It generally occurs in older age patients (greater than 50 years old).

C. Physical exam suggests a tender abdomen with rebound to the left lower quadrant, decreased bowel sounds, fever, tachycardia, tachypnea. Occasional mass in the involved area (diverticular abscess).

D. Pertinent laboratory will include elevated leukocyte count with left shift, hemo concentration and abdominal x-rays which are generally non-specific.

E. Treatment consists of NG suction, IV fluids, antibiotics and abdominal exploration to remove the offending portion of the colon and create a fecal diversion if symptoms don't rapidly improve.

IX. Small bowel obstruction (SBO)

A. SBO may be the cause of acute abdominal pain but is not commonly associated with acute sudden onset pain. Most common presentation is that of progressive abdominal distention with crampy colicky abdominal pain, associated with nausea, vomiting and obstipation.

B. Examination reveals a distended, tympanitic abdomen with high-pitched, active bowel sounds.

C. Laboratory reveals mildly elevated white cell count and hemo concentration on hemogram and electrolytes, abdominal x-rays reveal distended loops of small bowel in a stair step fashion with air fluid levels and no air in the colon.

D. Treatment consists of NG suction, IV fluids and hydration, usually prophylactic antibiotics and abdominal exploration after fluid resuscitation to prevent development of strangulation and bowel rupture.

X. Genitourinary problems

A. Urolithiasis

1. Sudden onset of abdominal or flank pain radiating toward testicle that is extremely severe. Patient often cannot find a position of comfort.

2.   Urinalysis reveals hematuria; 90% of renal stones show up on x-ray. IVP can be helpful.

3.   Treat with IV hydration and analgesics, occasionally retrieval with a basket in OR, or with lithotripsy.

B.   Testicular torsion

1.   Occurs in young men (< 25 year). Abrupt onset of severe pain with associated nausea and vomiting.

2.   Requires urgent operative intervention.

ESOPHAGUS

I.   Anatomic points of interest

    A.   Two layers striate muscle upper one-third, smooth muscle lower two-thirds.

    B.   Muscle with no serosa (= difficult to sew)

    C.   Squamous epithelium - columnar epithelium

    D.   No anatomic lower esophageal sphincter (LES) - physiologic only, relying on unique anatomic relationships.

    E.   Blood supply from aorta via direct and anastomosing branches

    F.   Lies in posterior mediastinum in chest - right side of midline, upper two-thirds; left side of midline in lower one-third.

II.   Physiology

    A.   General

        1.   Peristaltic wave - voluntary up high, then involuntary propagation

        2.   LES relaxes to accept food passage, then returns to normal resting pressure (15-25 cm H_2O above pressure in stomach).

        3.   Tertiary contractions in older patients

    B.   Assessment

1. Esophageal manometry

    a. Small catheter with pressure transducers at 5 cm intervals which track pressure wave through swallowing mechanism.

2. pH monitoring to evaluate reflux esophagitis.

    a. Same or similar catheter - pH in esophagus at various positions - check time to clearance of acid - may do 24 hour pH monitoring for number of reflux episodes and time to clearance of acid.

3. Bernstein provocative test - instill acid in esophagus to see if symptoms recur.

4. Barium swallow

III. Pathology

A. Motility disorders

1. Cricopharyngeal muscle dysfunction - Zenker's diverticula (post-midline) - pulsion type

    a. Symptoms of regurgitation, putrid breath odor.

    b. Treated with excision of redundant mucosa and myotomy.

2. Epiphrenic diverticula - often don't need treatment.

3. Achalasia - inability to relax LES - dilated esophagus - Bird's beak appearance -more dysphagia with liquid than solids. Rx with balloon dilatation or Heller myotomy.

4. "Nutcracker"esophagus - increased motility - chest pain - Rx NTG, nifedipine.

5. Presbyesophagus - tertiary contraction

6. Scleroderma - poor or no motility - difficulty swallowing, weight loss

B. Reflux esophagitis

1. Often associated with sliding hiatal hernias (Type I)

       a.   E-G junction moves into mediastinum.

    2.   Treatment of reflux esophagitis - elevate head of bed, antacids, +/- H2 blockers, discontinue ETOH, tobacco, caffeine.

    3.   Operate for intractable symptoms, bleeding, stricture (obstruction) - Nissen, Hill, Belsey - 80% + success.

    4.   Barrett's esophagus - columnar metaplasia of lower part of esophagus, due to chronic acid injury - increased incidence adenocarcinoma (10%).

C.   Paraesophageal hernias

    1.   Potential for incarceration, strangulation, ulcer with bleeding, perforation - repair when found.

    2.   E-G junction remains in place while stomach herniates through hiatus into mediastinum.

D.   Cancer

    1.   Associated with tobacco/ETOH abuse, diet, vitamin deficiency, poor oral hygiene, caustic burns, Barrett's esophagus, radiation and Plummer-Vinson syndrome.

    2.   Squamous cell carcinoma (SCC) in upper two-thirds.

    3.   Adenocarcinoma in lower one-third with upper gastric cancer.

    4.   Dysphagia with solids > liquids; weight loss.

    5.   SCC - some response to radiation and chemotherapy (Cisplatinum) - usually also excised.

    6.   Adenocarcinoma - minimal response to radiation/chemotherapy - excision.

    7.   Five year survival - low (5%).

STOMACH

I. **Anatomy**

    A. Fundus and body

        1. Parietal cells - HCL

        2. Chief cells - pepsinogen

    B. Antrum - G cells - gastrin

    C. Pylorus - controls rate of gastric emptying

    D. Arteries

        1. Left and right gastric (via celiac axis)

        2. Left and right gastroepiploic

        3. Short gastric branches

        4. Gastroduodenal

    E. Veins and lymphatics follow arteries

    F. Nerves

        1. Vagus enters via esophageal hiatus with the left trunk anterior (also supplies gallbladder and liver) and the right trunk posterior (also supplies mid-gut).

II. **Physiology**

A.   Digestive function

    1.   HCL and pepsinogen production stimulated by:

        a.   Cephalic - sight, smell, thought of food stimulates vagal release of histamine to increase HCL/pepsinogen (H2 receptors).

        b.   Gastric phase - gastric wall distention and presence of protein, etc, increases HCL secretion by stretch and stimulates gastrin release by G-cells which also increase HCL/pepsinogen secretion.

            (1)   Acid secretion also stimulated by ETOH, caffeine, tobacco, Ca^{++}

        c.   Intestinal phase - acidic contents and distention of small bowel cause decreased gastric motility and gastric acid/pepsin release by secretin. Secretin also stimulates gallbladder contraction and pancreas secretion.

    2.   Motility - gastric motility regulated by vagal innervation of H2 receptor sites.

III.   Diagnostic tools

A.   Radiography - barium swallow, upper gastrointestinal series (UGI) - easy, relatively cheap, 80-90% sensitivity/specificity.

B.   Endoscopy - flexible "EGD" esophagogastroduodenoscopy - very safe/accurate - can do biopsies.

C.   Acid analyses

    1.   Basal acid output

    2.   Maximum acid output - stimulated by histamine or pentagastrin; inhibited by secretin.

IV.   Peptic ulcer disease

A.   Associated factors - normal to high basal acid output, "Type A" personality, blood group A.

B.   Symptoms - burning epigastric pain on empty stomach (especially middle of night) - relieved with food or antacids.

1. Worse with caffeine, ETOH, various foods for various patients.

C. Diagnosis - UGI or EGD - most are in first portion of duodenum or in pylorus.

D. Treatment

    1. Most respond to pharmacologic acid reduction (90%) - H2 blockers (cimetidine, ranitidine, omeprazole) or antacids plus avoidance of high acid producing foods (ETOH, caffeine, CA++).

    2. Indications for operation - hemorrhage (> 6 units in 12 hours, re-bleed in hospital, visible artery in base of ulcer) perforation (25% don't have free air), gastric outlet obstruction and intractable symptoms in spite of good medical management.

    3. Operations include:

        a. Proximal gastric vagotomy (PGV) - 15% long-term recurrence but low complication (i.e., dumping, early satiety, loop syndromes, malabsorption syndromes, etc.)

        b. Selective vagotomy plus outlet procedure - essentially not done any more.

        c. Truncal vagotomy and pyloroplasty - 10% recurrence rate - minimal post-vagotomy syndromes.

        d. Truncal vagotomy, antrectomy, gastroduodenostomy (Billroth I) or gastrojejunostomy (Billroth II) have 1.5% recurrence rate (best) but increased incidence of dumping, afferent/efferent loop problems, etc.

V. Gastric ulcer disease

A. Associated factors

    1. Directed mucosal injury - ASA, steroids, ischemia associated with shock (stress ulcers), ETOH (gastritis).

    2. Low basal acid output, mucous barrier breakdown with re-diffusion H+ into cells, achlorhydria, type 0 blood group, blue collar economic class, increased Far East cultures.

    3. Gastric cancers

B.   Symptoms - epigastric pain - variable relief with food/antacids - weight loss.

C.   Diagnosis - UGI or EGD with biopsy - most are on lesser curve near antrum - beware of those on greater curve.

D.   Treatment

    1.   Antacids, H_2 blocks, cytoprotective agents (sucralfate, omeprazole) along with avoiding or correcting underlying mucosal injury agents are effective. Pharmacologic management has 50-60% recurrence rate for benign gastric ulcers.

        a.   Must re-endoscope or UGI series after six weeks to be sure ulcer has healed.

    2.   Indications for operation - hemorrhage, obstruction, perforation, or intractable, with best medical management (if ulcer not healed within 6 weeks, the ulcer needs to be excised to eliminate the possibility of cancer).

    3.   Operations include:

        a.   Excision of ulcer - antrectomy if ulcer is distal (the ulcer must be excised).

        b.   Vagotomy added if patient secretes significant acid.

VI.   Post-gastrectomy syndromes

A.   Early dumping

    1.   Uncontrolled dumping of hypertonic fluid into small bowel - results in acute hypovolemia and release of vasoactive hormones (serotonin, histamine, glucagon, VIP, etc).

    2.   Manifested by weakness, tachycardia, diaphoresis, palpitations and occasional diarrhea.

    3.   Treat by avoiding liquids with meals, avoid high CHO, ingest some fat with each meal and some recommended propranolol.

B.   Late dumping

    1.   Similar symptoms to early dumping but occurs 3-5 hours after meal.

2. Due to rapid changes in insulin and glucose levels.

3. Treated by eating a small snack two hours after meals.

C. Afferent loop obstruction

1. Occurs after Billroth II reconstruction and is associated with a kink in the afferent limb.

2. Build up of pancreatic and bile juice causes crampy pain and finally vomiting without food particles.

3. Treat with conversion of Billroth II to Roux-en-Y anastomosis.

D. Blind loop syndrome

1. Bacterial overgrowth in a loop or limb of bowel which does not have chyme flowing through it.

2. Interferes with folate and vitamin B_{12} metabolism leading to weakness and anemia.

3. Treat with antibiotics.

E. Alkaline reflux gastritis

1. Weakness, weight loss, nausea, abdominal pain and anemia due to reflux of alkaline biliary/pancreatic fluid into stomach.

2. Treatment - divert biliary fluid away from stomach.

F. Nutritional deficiencies

1. Especially vitamin B_{12}, folate, iron.

2. Many patients have diarrhea and weight loss.

VII. **Gastric cancer**

A. Adenocarcinoma most common - rare lymphoma, leiomyosarcoma, etc.

B. Associated factors same as with gastric ulcers - also achlorhydria, pernicious anemia, Barrett's esophagus, lye ingestion.

C.   Diagnosis - UGI/EGD with biopsy.

D.   Treatment - operative removal. Chemotherapy, radiation therapy not very helpful. Survival with operation < 10% 5 year due to advanced stage at diagnosis.

SMALL BOWEL

I.   Anatomy

    A.   Duodenum - 4 parts - from pylorus to ligament of Treitz; Brunner's glands.

        1.   Gastroduodenal artery and pancreatoduodenal arterial arcades

        2.   Ampulla of Vater (sphincter of Oddi)

    B.   Jejunum - central two thirds of bowel.

        1.   Superior mesenteric artery and vein (SMA & V)

    C.   Ileum - distal one third of small bowel

        1.   SMA & V

        2.   Meckel's diverticulum

            a.   Within 2 feet of ileocecal valve, antimesenteric border; two types of aberrant mucosa (gastric and pancreatic); common lead point of intussusception in 2 year olds.

        3.   Ileocecal valve

        4.   Peyer's patches - lymphatic collections

II. **Physiology**

    A. Absorption/Digestion

        1. Break down of proteins to polypeptides, fats to fatty acids, and complex carbohydrates (CHO) to simple sugars begins in duodenum with various enzymes (trypsin, chymotrypsin, elastase, lipase, amylase, etc.)

        2. Absorption occurs throughout remainder of bowel - proteins and CHO by active processes, lipids by passive diffusion.

        3. Ileum - specialized absorption of Fe (with intrinsic factor secreted by stomach), lipids and bile salts (enterohepatic circulation).

    B. Motility

        1. Parasympathetic innervation from vagus (X), increases tone and intestinal motility.

        2. Intrinsic motility is present in response to changes in intraluminal pressures.

        3. Sympathetic innervation slows tone and motility.

    C. Endocrine

        1. Multiple hormones including VIP, secretin, enterogastrone, etc.

        2. Trophic hormones for bowel mucosa growth.

III. **Crohn's Disease**

    A. Most common intrinsic disease of small bowel.

        1. Etiology unknown

        2. Increased incidence 2nd-3rd decade and 6-7th decade

        3. Non-caseating granulomatous inflammation of entire bowel wall

        4. Skip areas frequent - fissures in mucosa

        5. Most commonly involves terminal ileum; can involve any part of the bowel

6. May cause enteral fistulae

B. Manifestations

1. Crampy abdominal pain, low grade fever, bloody diarrhea, weight loss

2. May present like acute appendicitis

3. May present with persistent perianal disease - fistulae, fissures, abscesses

C. Diagnosis

1. Barium enema, UGI with small bowel follow through - "string"sign in distal ileum.

2. Colonoscopy/EGD if within reach of the instruments - cobblestoning, linear erosions/fissures.

D. Treatment

1. Azulfidine/prednisone for acute flare-ups. May need parenteral hyperalimentation.

2. Maintenance medication occasionally helpful with Azulfidine.

3. Surgical excision for:

a. hemorrhage

b. obstruction

c. perforation

d. intractable symptoms

4. Recurrence rate of approximately 50% in 8 years.

IV. Small bowel obstruction

A. Etiology

1. Postoperative adhesions (60%)

    2.   Incarceration in hernias (20%)

    3.   Others - Crohn's disease intussusception, volvulus, tumors

B.   Types of obstruction

    1.   Simple obstruction - most common

    2.   Closed loop obstruction - early necrosis and perforation with minimal prodromal illness (i.e., volvulus, etc.).

    3.   Partial obstruction - continues to pass gas and occasionally will resolve spontaneously.

    4.   Strangulated obstruction - bowel necrosis

C.   Diagnosis

    1.   History - nausea, vomiting, obstipation, crampy abdominal pain.

    2.   Physical exam - distended, tympanic abdomen, hyperactive bowel sounds.

    3.   X-ray - dilated loops small bowel, air-fluid levels, no gas in colon.

D.   Treatment

    1.   Fluid resuscitation

        a.   Correct isotonic fluid losses plus hypokalemic, hypochloremic metabolic alkalosis

    2.   NG decompression

    3.   Early laparotomy to relieve the obstruction.

E.   Differential diagnosis

Paralytic Ileus	**Small Intestinal Obstruction**
1. Minimal abdominal pain	1. Crampy abdominal pain
2. Nausea and vomiting	2. Nausea and vomiting

3. Obstipation and failure to pass flatus
4. Abdominal distension
5. Decreased or absent bowel sounds
6. Gas in the small intestine and colon on x-ray

3. Obstipation and failure to pass flatus
4. Abdominal distension
5. Normal or increased bowel sounds
6. Gas in the small intestine only on x-ray

V. **Small bowel cancers**

A. Adenocarcinoma most common, intrinsic cancer of SB (most common in duodenum).

1. Carcinoids in small bowel, second only to appendix.

a. Carcinoid syndrome - associated with liver metastasis - consists of episodes of serotonin surge, flushing, hyperperistalsis, diarrhea, bronchospasm, etc. (5HT)

2. Lymphoma also may involve small bowel.

3. Occasionally leiomyosarcoma, etc.

B. Signs/symptoms - primarily obstruction, also occasional bleeding.

C. Treatment of most tumors revolves around excision.

1. Lymphoma is responsive to chemotherapy.

APPENDIX

I.   **Inflammation**

    A.   Pathophysiology

        <u>Obstruction</u> of lumen (fecalith, extrinsic lymphatic obstruction, etc.), bacterial overgrowth and release of or activation of local vasoactive peptides, decreased absorptive capacity while mucosa continues to secrete, increased intramural pressure leading to compression of lymphatics, venules, and then arteriolar capillaries which leads to necrosis and perforation.

    B.   Diagnosis

        1.   History - most common in 2nd or 3rd decade - starts with vague periumbilical discomfort, mild nausea, fever, anorexia - pain subsequently localizes to right lower quadrant with local peritoneal irritation and signs.

        2.   Exam - tenderness near right lower quadrant (McBurney's point), normal bowel sounds, mild fever, right lower quadrant pain on rectal exam.

        3.   Lab - mild increased WBC, occasional WBC/RBC in urine, otherwise normal.

        4.   X-ray - occasional right lower quadrant fecalith

            a.   Barium enema not reliably helpful.

        5.   Negative surgical exploration in 20% is reasonable (35% in women during childbearing years).

    C.   Treatment - excision, open or through laparoscope

D. Differential diagnosis

1. Pelvic inflammatory disease - in women, look for tenderness with movement of cervix, bilateral pain, higher fever and WBC.

2. Crohn's disease - may present with clinical picture like acute appendicitis in 25% of patients. Diagnosis made by inspection of bowel at the time of exploration (creeping fat over serosa of small bowel; thick, shortened mesentery; prominent neovascularization).

3. Meckel's diverticulitis - urinary tract infection (with right pyelonephritis); ureteral stone disease; acute cholecystitis; perforated peptic ulcer disease; torsion of the testes; acute pancreatitis; gastroenteritis; etc.

E. Groups at high risk for perforation

1. Neonates - disease is rare in this age because appendix is a short, broad-based diverticulum and the very young do not have much lymphatic tissue in walls of the appendix to cause obstruction.

2. Pregnant patients - delay in diagnosis of appendicitis and reluctance to treat; abnormal location of the appendix and the pain associated with it; inability of the omentum to reach the site of inflammation and contain the process.

3. Elderly - delay in diagnosis and treatment; low level of suspicion in elderly patients; signs and symptoms are often not as specific as in younger patients.

II. **Neoplasias**

A. Carcinoid tumor - unusual but most common tumor of appendix

1. Small-cell neuroendocrine (chromaffin cell) cell line origin

2. Found in appendix (50%), rectum, ileum, lungs

3. Metastasizes to liver then becomes symptomatic due to release of serotonin - measured as 5-HT in urine.

4. Primary treatment is excision if < 2 cm; right hemicolectomy if > 2 cm. Anti-serotonin agents will help control symptoms.

B. Adenocarcinoma - unusual mass lesion of the appendix; has the histology and prognosis of adenocarcinoma of the colon; diagnosis rarely made prior to excision of mass found incidentally.

C.   Lymphoma - unusual

      1.   Treated like other visceral lymphomas

COLON

I. Introduction

A. Anatomy

1. Ileocecal valve - cecum - right colon - hepatic flexure - transverse colon - splenic flexure - descending colon - sigmoid colon.

2. Three longitudinal tinea divide the colon into thirds - vertical incomplete haustra formed by muscular bands that partake in peristalsis.

3. Arterial supply from superior mesenteric artery to ileocolic artery, right colic artery and middle colic artery. Left colon supplied by branches of the inferior mesenteric artery - left colic artery and superior hemorrhoidals. Arterial supply connects through marginal artery of Drummond and the meandering artery of Riolan.

4. Venous and lymphatic systems generally follow the arterial patterns.

B. Physiology

1. Tremendous ability to conserve water and electrolytes by absorption.

2. Involuntary peristaltic waves move stool through colon - "mass movement".

3. Serves as a vital storage organ.

II. Neoplastic diseases

A. Polyps

1.   Juvenile polyps - may cause bleeding in children; usually self-limited; no malignant potential.

2.   Hamartomas - seen with Peutz-Jeghers syndrome; is associated with melanin spots on lips; no malignant potential.

3.   Tubular adenomas - most common type of polyp found; usually small (< 0.5 cm); low malignant potential (5% associated with cancers) unless numerous or large (> 1 cm).

    a.   Familial polyposis - autosomal dominant disease of thousands of tubular adenomatous polyps in colon; usually found in 2nd decade of life in susceptible families; risk of cancer is virtually 100% unless colon removed prophylactically (usually done as total abdominal colectomy, rectal mucosectomy, ileoanal pouch anastomosis to retain continence).

    b.   Gardner's syndrome - tubular adenomas throughout GI tract (although not as numerous as familial polyposis); associated with exostosis (esp. maxilla) and inclusion cysts in skin; - moderate malignant potential.

4.   Villotubular adenomas - histologic picture of both tubular and villous elements; less common than tubular adenomas but higher association with malignancy (approximately 20%).

5.   Villous adenomas - more unusual than villotubular adenomas but higher malignant potential (approximately 35%) especially if larger (> 3 cm). May cause a syndrome of watery diarrhea with huge loses of KCL resulting in hypokalemia.

B.   Adenocarcinoma of colon

1.   Most common visceral cancer in United States - behind only lung and breast as cause of cancer deaths.

2.   Etiology unknown - thought to be related to dietary habits high in animal fats and low in fiber. Higher association with various polyps, ulcerative colitis, Crohn's colitis and lymphogranuloma venereum.

3.   More common in left and sigmoid colon (50-70%)

    a.   Synchronous tumors in 5%

        b.   Metachronous tumors 3-5%.

4. Left sided tumors tend to develop into constricting "apple-core"lesions resulting in symptoms of "constipation",pencil-thin stools, occult blood with occasional bright red blood, partial or total bowel obstruction.

5. Right sided tumors tend to develop into polypoid, fungating masses which cause anemia and inanition resulting in fatigue, weight loss, poor appetite, occult blood in stool, etc.

6. Both are diagnosed by colonoscopy with biopsy or barium enema. 5% incidence of synchronous lesions (other tumors present at the same time but different place).

7. Treatment involves removal of tumor bearing colon, along with wide margins of normal colon and the lymphatic drainage bed.

8. Prognosis is most related to lymphatic involvement and metastatic spread - various modification of Duke's classification scheme are used.

        a.   Disease limited to mucosa, 80-90% 5 year survival.

        b.   Disease through wall of colon, no lymph node or distant spread, 60-70% 5 year survival.

        c.   Disease involves lymph nodes, 30% 5 year survival.

        d.   Distant metastases, < 5% 5 year survival.

9. Isolated metastases to liver can be removed with improved long-term survival.

10. Various large scale screening efforts to detect the cancer earlier (including proctoscopy, fecal occult blood testing, CEA antigen levels in serum) have been largely unrewarding.

11. Chemotherapy for metastatic disease has had limited success; radiation therapy has not been helpful except in reducing the bulk of large rectal cancers.

III. Inflammatory diseases

    A.   Diverticulitis

1.	Diverticula are mucosal hernias through the muscularis and occur at points in the colon where end arteries enter the bowel wall; are thought to be related to diets low in fiber/bulk - they occur in most people in Western cultures who live long enough - present in up to 70% of elderly patients, more common in left colon.

2.	Erosion into an adjacent artery, without inflammation, may lead to massive blood loss (diverticulosis).

3.	Obstruction of the lumen of a diverticulum leads to bacterial overgrowth, swelling, inflammation and possibly to rupture and abscess formation - "diverticulitis".

4.	Presentation is like a "left-sided"appendicitis in older patients.

5.	Treatment of mild cases involves antibiotics against coliforms, high bulk, high fiber diet, hydration. Cases involving intractable symptoms or repeated episodes, hemorrhage, obstruction due to stricture formation or perforation may need surgical removal of the diseased colon.

B.	Ulcerative colitis

1.	Inflammatory process of colonic mucosa and submucosa of unknown etiology; usually appears in 2nd - 3rd decade, but a second peak incidence around age 55.

2.	Signs and symptoms - crampy abdominal pain, bloody mucous diarrhea, often with fever, weight loss, fatigue, etc. Clinical picture varies from occasional flare-ups (55% of patients) to acute fulminant illness with massive dilation of colon and sepsis (15% of patients) (toxic megacolon). Usual process is repeated episodes of illness with cramps, bloody diarrhea and associated symptoms.

3.	Diagnosis is usually with colonoscopy (erosion of mucosa with "pseudopolyps"covers large areas, no skip areas) or barium enema during quiescent phases (foreshortening of colon, loss of haustra, "lead pipe" appearance).

4.	Symptoms can often be controlled (80%) with systemic steroids, Azulfidine and motility inhibitors (codeine).

5.	Long term risk includes increased risk of cancer - 4% at 10 years and cancer risk increased by approximately 2% per year thereafter. Greater amount of colon involved and greater activity of the disease leads to even greater cancer risk.

6. Disease is cured by removal of all colon mucosa - usually done as total colectomy, rectal mucosectomy, ileoanal reservoir anastomosis.

IV. Large bowel obstruction

A. Colon cancer (65%)

B. Diverticular disease (20%)

C. Volvulus (5%) - sigmoid followed by cecal - more common in older, nursing home patients with poor colonic function - long mesentery which allows twisting of the involved segment. Diagnosis with plain x-rays of abdomen. Sigmoid volvulus occasionally relieved with rectal tube but often recurs, requiring removal of redundant sigmoid. Cecal volvulus usually treated with cecopexy if bowel wall viability not in question.

D. Pseudo-obstruction - (Ogilvie's syndrome) dilated portion of colon - usually transverse and right side without mechanical lesion; usually in older patients often on digoxin and anti-Parkinson medications.

E. Treatment of colon obstruction usually requires colostomy and removal of offending portion with reanastomosis done separately after the colon can be prepped.

V. Lower GI hemorrhage

A. Melena

1. Source can be anywhere in GI tract - requires only approximately 50 cc's blood to create guaiac positive stools.

2. Most common source of melena is UGI bleed, therefore investigate esophagus, stomach, duodenum first.

3. Sources below ligament of Treitz include small bowel tumors (polyps or cancers), Meckel's diverticulum, Crohn's disease, A-V malformations, diverticulosis of the colon (most common source, approximately 70%), colon cancers, small bowel or colon ischemia and ulcerative colitis.

4. Management includes fluid resuscitation, restoration of clotting factors and search for etiology.

5. EGD, colonoscopy and arteriography are most useful diagnostic tools. Labelled RBC nuclear scans are occasionally helpful.

6. Surgical exploration without a diagnosis or location of bleeding preoperatively is often unrewarding.

B. Hematochezia - bright red blood per rectum

1. Consider diverticulosis, colonic telangiectasia (A-V malformations), hemorrhoids, colon cancers.

2. May occasionally occur with massive upper GI bleed.

RECTUM AND ANUS

I. **Rectum and anus**

   A. Anatomy

      1. Differs from remainder of colon in not having a serosal layer. Rectum lies outside peritoneal lining from peritoneal reflection to dentate line.

      2. Arterial supply from IMA via superior hemorrhoids and from internal iliacs via middle and inferior hemorrhoidal arteries. Venous and lymphatic drainage follow arterial supply.

      3. Outer external sphincter of striated, voluntary muscle and inner smooth, involuntary muscle.

   B. Physiology

      1. Intricate neuromuscular involvement in fecal continence - lower rectum/anus - external and internal sphincters plus puborectalis sling and levator ani.

   C. Adenocarcinoma - similar histologically with adenocarcinoma of colon with similar staging and prognosis schemes.

      1. Because of tendency to invade side walls of pelvis, radiation therapy pre or postoperative removal is sometimes helpful.

   D. Inflammatory disease

      1. Crohn's disease and ulcerative colitis both commonly involve the rectum - diagnosis and treatment is as described above.

2. Other inflammatory conditions include various infectious etiologies and radiation induced proctitis.

II. Anus

A. Anatomy/Physiology

1. Squamous epithelium blends to columnar mucosa at dentate line. Columns of Morgagni between crypts of Lieberkuhn secrete mucous, etc.

2. External and internal sphincters control continence and differentiate gas from stool.

B. Congenital problems

1. Imperforate anus - involves short or long segments of obliterated anus/rectum - requires immediate attention.

2. Hirschsprung's disease - lack of myomesenteric nerve bodies (Auerbach and Meissner) leading to poor colonic emptying and an abnormal constricted distal segment of anus/rectum/sigmoid/colon.

C. Inflammatory lesions

1. Peri-rectal abscess - obstructed mucous glands at dentate line resulting in an abscess which necessitates to the skin or occasionally will penetrate the sphincteric muscles to invade the ischial space; treated by incision and drainage.

2. Peri-anal fistulae often develop after drainage of a peri-rectal abscess; Goodsall's rule - cutaneous openings posterior to a horizontal line through the anus usually connect to a posterior midline internal opening, while cutaneous openings anterior to that line generally run directly straight to a mucosal opening; treated by opening the tract widely and debriding granulation tissue. (Recurrent lesions could be Crohn's disease).

3. Anal fissures - very painful superficial erosions in anterior or posterior midline, associated with constipation, especially in children; treated with dilation or internal sphincterotomy.

4. Perianal warts (condylomata acuminate) - viral etiology, are the most common.

D. Hemorrhoids

    1. Represent dilated veins - external ones are painful, may prolapse and thrombose or bleed. Internal hemorrhoids are not painful but cause bright red blood on tissue or outside of stool.

    2. Most can be treated with local anti-inflammatory agents, local pain suppressants, diet to reduce strain and constipation (increase fluids, increase bulk, stool softeners, etc) and Sitz baths.

    3. Thrombosed hemorrhoids, excessive bleeding, severe prolapse; all should be excised.

E. Neoplasia

    1. Epidermoid carcinoma is most common - usually presents as mass lesion, occasionally as fistula that won't heal.

    2. Tends to spread into surrounding soft tissues and femoral/iliac nodes.

    3. Reasonably responsive to radiation therapy.

    4. Cloacal carcinoma - unusual, squamous adenocarcinoma, often presents as a submucosal nontender mass. Generally poor prognosis.

    5. Malignant melanoma may occur in anus - treated like other melanomas.

GALLBLADDER AND BILIARY SYSTEM

I.   Anatomy

    A.   Common bile duct (empties through ampulla of Vater) - cystic duct (lined with valves of Heister) - common hepatic ducts - right and left hepatic ducts.

    B.   Common hepatic artery (from celiac axis) - gastroduodenal artery and proper hepatic artery - cystic artery.

    C.   Venous drainage and lymphatics follow arterial supply (Calot's node at bifurcation of cystic duct).

    D.   Ductal and arterial anatomy is <u>extremely variable</u>.

II.   Physiology

    A.   Serves as a storage and concentrating organ of liver-produced bile (500-1200 ml/day) - no untoward effects of not having a gallbladder.

    B.   Bile in gallbladder is a balance of the concentration of bile salts, (75%) phospholipids (lecithin) (20%) and cholesterol (5%) - abnormalities in this balance are part of development of stones.

    C.   Contraction stimulated by cholecystokinin (CCK) released from duodenum in response to fats and acidity. (CCK = pancreozymen)

III.   Congenital problems

    A.   Biliary atresia

        1.   Varying degrees of atresia of the extrahepatic and intrahepatic ducts with

prognosis inversely proportional to the degree of atresia.

2. Previously treated with biliary-enteric anastomoses; now treated with liver transplants when organs available.

IV. Calculus associated illnesses

A. Composition

1. May be pure "pigment stones" (25%) (bile salts, especially associated with hemolytic disorders, i.e., sickle cell anemia, spherocytosis, etc.), may be pure cholesterol stones (most responsive to dissolution therapy), but most commonly are "mixed stones" - pigment, cholesterol, calcium, etc.

B. Asymptomatic stones

1. Incidence of developing symptoms is approximately 20% over lifetime; once symptoms develop they usually recur.

2. High risk patients with asymptomatic stones (diabetes mellitus, immunosuppressed, etc.) should have gallbladder out before symptoms appear.

C. Acute cholecystitis

1. Inflammatory condition of gallbladder associated with stones > 90%.

2. Results from obstruction of cystic duct by stone, bacterial overgrowth with altered mucous membrane permeability, increased secretion versus absorption, swelling of gallbladder and edema of wall, leading to congestion of lymphatic, venous and then arterial flow (resulting in necrosis/perforation/gangrene).

a. Biliary colic represents repeated symptomatic episodes which spontaneously resolve (presumably because of migration of the obstructing stone).

3. Clinical manifestations

a. More common in overweight, middle aged, females.

b. Right upper quadrant crampy pain 30 minutes after meals heavy with greasy, fatty, spicy foods.

      c.   No reliable relief with antacids.

      d.   Associated with nausea, vomiting and occasionally fever.

      e.   15% of gallstones show up on plain x-ray.

      f.   Ultrasound very accurate at diagnosis.

      g.   Associated lab findings include increased WBC, increased alkaline phosphatase, only mildly increased bilirubin, mildly increased hepatocellular enzymes.

4.   Initial management includes NG suction, IV fluid resuscitation, antibiotics (cephalosporins are highly concentrated in bile - usual organisms include E. coli, Klebsiella, Enterobacter, Salmonella) and analgesics.

5.   Operative cholecystectomy (open or laparoscopic) urgently if symptoms don't abate or electively once symptoms are better.

6.   Approximately 5% will have unsuspected common duct stones found by palpation or on intraoperative cholangiograms and require common duct exploration.

D.   Chronic cholecystitis

1.   Signs, symptoms, pathophysiology are similar to acute cholecystitis. Patients have repeated, short, often self-limited bouts of biliary colic. Incidence of recurrence is very high.

2.   Treatment options

      a.   Operative removal of gallbladder - (open or laparoscopic) is treatment of choice.

      b.   Dissolution therapy - use of chenodeoxycholic acid to dissolve the 30-40% of stones which are pure cholesterol - requires months to work - high incidence of stone reformation with cessation of therapy - numerous complications of treatment, especially nausea and diarrhea.

      c.   Lithotripsy - use of directed ultrasound (either extracorporal, trans-common duct catheter or laser) to burst the stones - followed by dissolution therapy - expensive equipment, high incidence of

dissolution therapy - expensive equipment, high incidence of recurrence, potential for duct, liver, pancreas injury.

E. Choledocholithiasis

1. 15% of patients with gallstones will have stones in the common bile duct.

2. Right upper quadrant pain with jaundice and fever (Charcot's triad) is associated with acute descending cholangitis which represents a surgical emergency.

3. Diagnostic workup of jaundice associated with probable choledocholithiasis includes:

   a. Ultrasound

   b. Percutaneous transhepatic cholangiography (PTC)

   c. Endoscopic retrograde cholangiopancreatography (ERCP)

4. In the patient with Charcot's triad, urgent antibiotic therapy and drainage of the biliary tree, either by percutaneous placement of a catheter or operative opening of the common bile duct, is important to prevent death from overwhelming sepsis.

5. The patients with a symptomatic common bile duct stone, require operative removal.

   a. The absolute indications for exploring a common bile duct include a palpable common duct stone or common duct stones visualized on intraoperative cholangiogram.

   b. Relative indications include bile duct dilatation, jaundice, history of gallstone pancreatitis, multiple small stones and a single, multifaceted gallstone.

6. After exploration of the common bile duct, postoperative drainage through a T-tube is important because of a small chance of residual stones after exploration.

7. The operative mortality to cholecystectomy and common bile duct exploration may be as much as 8-10 percent.

F.   Gallstone associated pancreatitis

    1.   Second leading cause of acute pancreatitis in United States.

    2.   Occurs when a stone passes through ampulla of Vater, causing edema of orifice of pancreatic duct when pancreas is actively secreting. Usually do <u>not</u> find an impacted stone in the duct but can find stones in the stool.

    3.   Clinical manifestations similar to acute cholecystitis but with elevated serum amylase and epigastric, boring pain to the back.

    4.   Requires surgical removal of gallbladder and any common duct stones during same hospitalization after amylase has decreased and patient has resolved clinical symptoms.

G.   Gallstone ileus

    1.   Small bowel obstruction caused by a large gallstone which has eroded into duodenum (or occasionally jejunum) and becomes lodged in the small bowel (usually distal ileum).

    2.   Requires removal of the stone and gallbladder as well as repair of the biliary-enteric fistula.

V.   **Cancer**

A.   Common bile duct

    1.   Adenocarcinoma may occur in any area of the bile duct but most commonly involves the extrahepatic ducts. Etiology unknown, but associated with stones in 60%.

        a.   Other diseases associated with increased incidence of bile duct cancers include choledochal cysts, Charcot's disease and ulcerative colitis.

    2.   Patients are usually older (50, 60, 70's) and present with weight loss and painless, obstructive jaundice.

    3.   If ultrasound of liver reveals dilated ducts, percutaneous transhepatic cholangiography (PTC) helps determine whether the tumor is high (i.e. Klatskin's tumor at ductal bifurcation) or low (near the ampulla) and thus, the feasibility of operative intervention. CT scan can also help identify

intrahepatic lesions and metastasis to nearby lymph nodes. Occasionally ERCP will be able to see tumor and biopsy it.

4. Treatment is total excision, if possible, (often requiring a Whipple procedure) 10% operative mortality or palliation of obstructed ducts with bypass operation or stents if cure seems unlikely. Total removal carries a 30-40% 5 year survival. Chemotherapy and radiation are not very effective at this time.

B. Adenocarcinoma of gallbladder

1. Very unusual tumor, usually found at the time of cholecystectomy because of difficulty in dissecting the gallbladder from the liver bed. (80% are associated with gallstones)

2. Not sensitive to radiation or chemotherapy, so wide local excision is the treatment of choice with good, long term prognosis if tumor completely removed. Usually, however, tumor has metastasized before detection, leading to an overall 5 year survival of < 5%.

3. Calcification of gallbladder wall (porcelain gallbladder) has a 60% association with gallbladder cancer.

LIVER

I. Anatomy

A. Right lobe with (5) segments divided from left lobe (3 segments) through the bed of the gallbladder. (Falciform ligament divides medial from central segment of left lobe). Caudate and quadrate lobes are situated centrally.

B. Portal vein (formed from the confluence of the splenic and superior mesenteric veins) enters the liver at the hilum and disperses into the portal triads (along with the hepatic artery branches and bile duct branches). Portal vein supplies 75% of hepatic blood flow but 50% of O_2 delivery.

C. Hepatic artery (branch of celiac axis) supplies only 25% of blood flow but 50% of O_2 delivery via the portal triads.

D. Bile ducts in portal triads collect the secretions of the hepatocytes and confluences eventually leading to the right and left hepatic ducts, the proper hepatic duct and then the common bile duct.

E. Blood from the portal triad vessels (portal vein and hepatic artery) percolates past the Kupffer's cells (phagocytosis of foreign bodies, bacteria, etc.) down the columns of hepatocytes into the central vein. The central veins converge and eventually lead to the right, middle and left hepatic veins which drain into the inferior vena cava.

II. Physiology

A. Performs hemopoietic function in fetus and neonate.

B. Complex hepatocellular functions serve to metabolize numerous drugs and chemicals in the body as well as serving an immunosuppressive function of phagocytosis and entrapment. This includes detoxifying numerous metabolic by-products of normal GI function.

C.   Bile is formed as a breakdown product of hemoglobin. The enterohepatic circulation in which bile salts are reabsorbed in the terminal ileum is important for fatty acid absorption.

III.   Congenital abnormalities

A.   Most surgically important congenital hepatic problems involve atresia of the biliary tract and are covered in that chapter.

B.   Numerous congenital or genetic abnormalities of hepatic function may lead to the need for hepatic transplant, including Gauche's disease, Wilson's disease, etc.

IV.   Inflammatory problems

A.   Bacterial

1.   Non-traumatic bacterial infections of the liver are unusual.

2.   Pyogenic hepatic abscesses gain access to the liver via the biliary or portal venous system; most commonly involve enteric bacilli (E. coli, Klebsiella, Serratia, Salmonella, etc.) and originate with cholangitis, appendicitis, diverticulitis or occasionally salpingitis.

3.   Plain films of the abdomen may show air fluid levels in the liver of a patient with fever, right upper quadrant pain, +/- jaundice and suggest the diagnosis. CT scans and U/S are useful in localizing abscesses as well.

4.   In addition to treating the source of infection, intrahepatic abscesses should be drained if possible either operatively or now more commonly through percutaneously placed catheters, and treated with appropriate antibiotics, mortality 10-40%.

B.   Amebic abscesses

1.   Eosinophilia may accompany increased WBC, fever, etc.

2.   Usually can be treated with antibiotics with good results (Metronidazole).

3.   "Anchovy paste"-like material in cavity.

4. Occurs without amebic dysentery in 50% of cases.

C. Echinococcus cyst

1. Unusual - usually accompanies concomitant pulmonary disease - usually solitary, often calcified cyst in right lobe of liver.

2. Eosinophilia present.

3. Attempt to sterilize cyst by injection of hypertonic saline prior to excision or external drainage.

4. Important to avoid intra-abdominal spread.

D. Sclerosing cholangitis

1. Usually presents in 3rd - 4th decade as sepsis problems related to multiple intra-hepatic abscesses.

2. ERCP reveals multiple sclerotic bile ducts (intra - and extra-hepatic) with numerous abscess cavities in both lobes of the liver.

3. Etiology is thought to be autoimmune (associated with ulcerative colitis, etc.) but exact mechanism has not been determined.

4. Treatment involves drainage of abscesses, antibiotics and transplantation when possible.

V. **Portal hypertension**

A. Etiology

1. Pre-hepatic - portal vein occlusion (common in infants and children) or splenic vein occlusion (usually secondary to pancreatitis or trauma), associated with normal liver functions.

2. Intra-hepatic - ETOH induced cirrhosis most common in United States, also, post-hepatitis (post-necrotic) cirrhosis and intra-hepatic infections or metabolic problems which lead to obstruction of portal venous flow directly or indirectly via scarring (cirrhosis).

3. Post-hepatic - hepatic vein occlusion (Budd-Chiari syndrome) due to hypercoagulable state or tumor growth and obstruction of hepatic veins

(hypernephroma) associated with severe ascites.

4. Collateral venous decompression of elevated portal pressures occurs through 1) coronary vein/esophageal varices, 2) peri-umbilical veins (Caput Medusa), 3) superior hemorrhoidals, 4) veins of Retzius and 5) veins of Sappey.

B. Clinical manifestations and management

1. Upper GI bleeding due to enlarged esophageal or gastric varices is the most common manifestation.

   a. 75% of patients will re-bleed in one year and 60% will die in one year.

   b. Initial treatment includes IV fluid and coagulation defect correction, gastric lavage, IV Pitressin, esophagogastric balloon tamponade (Sengstaken-Blakemore tube).

   c. Early endoscopy and sclerotherapy effective in stopping initial hemorrhage in 85-90%.

   d. Long term management includes repeat sclerotherapy at regular intervals (problems with ulceration, stricture and development of gastric varices), portosystemic shunts (portocaval or mesocaval H-grafts) (5-10% perioperative mortality, 5% re-bleed rate, 20-30% encephalopathy rate), selective shunting (distal splenorenal shunt - 5% perioperative mortality, 10% re-bleed rate, 5% encephalopathy rate), TIPSS procedures (transjugular intrahepatic portosystemic shunt), and liver transplantation.

e. Perioperative prognosis predicted on basis of hepatic function. Child's classification

	A	B	C
Bilirubin	< 2.0	2.0 - 3.0	> 3.0
Albumin	> 3.5	3.0 - 3.5	< 3.0
Ascites	None	Easily controlled	Not easily controlled
Enceph	None	Minimum	Advanced
Nutrition	Excellent	Good	Poor
Mortality	**5%**	**10%**	**40%**

2. Ascites is due to increased perfusion pressure required to move blood from portal vein through hepatocyte columns to hepatic veins, resulting in leakage of high protein fluid into lymphatics and through liver capsule into peritoneal space. Formation further aggravated due to hemodilution from secondary hyperaldosteronism due to poor aldosterone metabolism by the sick liver.

a. Ascites usually a very prominent feature of patients with hepatic vein occlusion (Budd-Chiari) and often of patients with intra-hepatic cirrhosis, but ascites does not generally form in patients with portal vein occlusion.

b. Most ascites can be controlled with bed rest, sodium restriction and gentle diuresis (Spironolactone). Peritoneal - venous shunts can be helpful but can thrombose or induce a consumptive coagulopathy or lead to pulmonary edema. Portosystemic shunts (portocaval or mesocaval) are occasionally done to relieve severe ascites.

3. Encephalopathy is thought to be due to inadequate hepatic metabolism of toxic substances in the blood. The degree of encephalopathy varies from mild forgetfulness through to hepatic coma and has been loosely related to arterial ammonia level and more closely related to spinal glutamine levels.

a. Usual treatment includes dietary protein restriction, clearance of blood from GI tract, lactulose to inhibit ammonia production by enteric bacterial treatment of any concomitant infection.

VI. Neoplasias

A. Benign

1. Hepatic adenomas (associated with birth control pills), focal nodular hyperplasia and hemangiomas are the most common.

2. These usually do not require any treatment unless they grow to very large size, rupture, or cause pain, in which cases they are removed.

B. Malignant

1. Most common malignancy in liver is metastatic disease from other primary sites; especially colon.

2. Resection of isolated metastatic lesions (especially from colon carcinoma) can increase survival.

3. Primary hepatomas are relatively unusual in USA but more common in Oriental populations.

    a. Three main types are hepatoma, cholangiocarcinoma or mixed type.

        (1) Related to cirrhosis, hepatitis B, alpha-1 antitrypsin deficiency, hemochromatosis.

    b. Diagnosis can be made when a tender hepatic mass is identified on exam, localized by CT and often evaluated for possible resection with arteriogram.

    c. Treatment involves resection when possible. These tumors are fairly resistant to chemotherapy and radiation therapy.

PANCREAS

I. Anatomy

A. Two embryonic buds come together during gut alignment to yield one gland - main pancreatic duct of Wirsung - minor duct of Santorini.

B. Bounded on right by duodenum, left by spleen, anteriorly by stomach and transverse mesocolon and posteriorly by common bile duct, aorta, IVC, SMA/V.

C. Arterial supply from gastroduodenal artery, splenic artery and gastroepiploic arteries. Venous and lymphatic drainage basically follow arterial routes.

D. Histologic anatomy includes ductal cells, acini cells and islets of Langerhans.

II. Physiology

A. Exocrine

1. Stimulus of fat, protein and acid in duodenum cause secretion of 1000-5000 ml/d of pH8 fluid, chymotrypsinogen, trypsinogen, lipase, amylase, carboxypeptidase - all for digestion of proteins, carbohydrates and fats.

2. CCK-PZ and secretin are released from duodenal mucosa in response to amino acids, fats or acid. CCK increases the enzymes in pancreatic juice; Secretin stimulates flow of HCO_3-rich water and electrolytes.

B. Endocrine

1.   Includes insulin (beta cells), glucagon (alpha cells), gastrin (delta cells) and others.

III.   Inflammatory conditions

A.   Acute pancreatitis

1.   Most commonly related to ETOH (40%) - induced ductal and parenchymal cell injury.

2.   Also commonly associated with passage of gallstones past ampulla of Vater.

3.   Other etiologies include trauma, hypertriglyceridemia medications, (HCTA, steroids, lasix, estrogens) Type I, IV and V hyperlipoproteinemia, familial and postoperative ischemia.

4.   Manifested by epigastric abdominal pain boring through to back, with fever, nausea, vomiting and elevated serum amylase and lipase levels.

    a.   Cullen's sign (periumbilical hematoma) or Grey-Turner's sign (flank hematoma) suggests hemorrhagic pancreatitis.

5.   Initial treatment includes NG suction, IV fluids, nutrition, analgesia and possibly somatostatin to decrease exocrine function.

    a.   Surgery usually reserved for complications.

6.   Complications include:

    a.   Pancreatic necrosis and abscess - manifested by fever, increased WBC and persistent pain, gas on abdominal x-ray or CT scan. Requires drainage, antibiotics and nutrition.

    b.   Pseudocyst - due to leakage of a pancreatic duct and manifested by continued pain and mass. Those below 2 cm often resolve spontaneously. Larger ones or those that don't resolve are allowed to "mature" for 6 weeks and then internally drained into the stomach or a Roux-en-Y limb of jejunum. Has a fibrous lining vs. epithelium.

    c.   Pancreatic ascites - leakage of ductal contents into abdominal cavity; does not respond to usual treatment of ascites; needs internal drainage.

d. Hemorrhagic pancreatitis - erosion into surrounding vessels can lead to pseudoaneurysms, massive bleeding or massive retroperitoneal bleeding and necrosis.

e. Other complications include pancreatic fistulae, pulmonary insufficiency, eventual pancreatic endocrine and/or exocrine dysfunction, etc.

7. Prognosis of acute pancreatitis is best estimated by Ranson's criteria (which do not include level of serum amylase)!

a. Ranson's criteria

At admission: age > 55; WBC > 16K; glucose > 200; LDH > 350; SGOT > 250. During 48 hours after admission: Hct > 10 point decrease; BUN > 5 increase; Ca^{++} < 8.0; pO_2 < 60 mmHg room air; base excess > 4 mEq/l; est. fluid sequestration > 6000 mL.

b. Mortality 20% with 3-4 signs; 40% with 5-6 signs; 100% if 7 or more signs.

B. Chronic pancreatitis

1. Similar etiology to acute pancreatitis but marked by endocrine/exocrine dysfunction (diabetes mellitus/steatorrhea) and calcifications in pancreas on abdominal x-rays.

2. Chronic pain syndrome is investigated with ERCP and treated with internal drainage of dilated obstructed ducts (sphincterotomy or Peustow pancreatojejunostomy) or pancreatic resection if preservation of pancreatic function no longer an issue.

IV. **Neoplasia**

A. Non islet cell

1. Ductal adenocarcinoma is most common - often multicentric, associated with cigarette smoking and perhaps ETOH.

2. May occur at any location in pancreas - those in tail and body (1/3) are often far advanced prior to any symptoms. Those in the head (2/3) often

lead to painless obstructive jaundice.

3.   Evaluate with CT scans, PTC, ERCP as needed.

4.   Treated with excision when possible with 5% five year survival in the 10-20% which can be resected for cure (Whipple procedure). Not very responsive to chemotherapy or radiation treatment.

5.   Cyst adenocarcinoma may mimic pseudocyst but has an epithelial lining and requires total excision.

B.   Islet cell tumors

1.   Gastrinoma, insulinoma, VIPoma and other functional tumors of APUD cell deviation.

2.   Gastrinoma associated with Zollinger-Ellison syndrome of hyperacidity, unresponsive to further acid output stimulation, resulting in diffuse peptic ulceration in stomach, duodenum and occasionally small bowel.

    a.   Marked by increased basal acid output, no increase in acid with stimulation, increased serum gastrin levels, paradoxic decrease in gastrin with IV secretin (secretin stimulation test).

    b.   Associated with MEN-I syndrome (pituitary and parathyroid adenomas).

    c.   Tumors from delta cells are often very small and may be multicentric but are not usually histologically malignant.

    d.   If symptoms are not controlled with H_2 blockers, laparotomy indicated to try to remove tumor or do PGV to relieve symptoms. Severe or recurrent disease usually treated with total gastrectomy.

3.   Insulinoma - associated with Whipple triad of symptoms of hypoglycemia, with fasting low blood sugar (< 50 mg%) and relief of symptoms with glucose. Have inappropriately high insulin levels.

    a.   Caused by a benign adenoma, occasionally localized with CT scan, MR or arteriography.

    b.   On-line blood glucose determinations helpful during resection to assure removal of the tumor.

4.   VIPomas - Vasointestinal peptides - neuroendocrine derived tumor causing a watery diarrhea, flushing, tachycardia syndrome. Relieved by tumor excision.

SPLEEN

I. **Anatomy**

    A.   Usually one lobe but may have lobulations - maintained by four suspensory ligaments.

    B.   Accessory spleens are congenital masses of splenic tissue with blood supply derived from splenic vessels. Present in 15-30% of patients.

    C.   Splenosis is bits of splenic tissue embedded in the omentum or mesentery as a result of splenic injury.

    D.   Histologic architecture involves red pulp (primary vascular) and white pulp (primary lymph tissue) with a portal venous system.

    E.   Main arterial supply from splenic artery but also branches from left gastroepiploic arteries.

    F.   Venous drainage includes splenic vein (with numerous pancreatic branches) and short gastric veins.

    G.   Pancreas, stomach, adrenal and left kidney are all very close anatomically and can be injured during splenic operations.

II. **Function logic**

    A.   Hematologic

        1.   Spleen makes RBCs and WBCs in fetus (5th to 8th month) until bone marrow matures.

2. Spleen clears blood stream of senescent RBCs and other cellular debris by phagocytosis.

B. Immunologic

1. Spleen aids B-cell antibody formation in response to foreign proteins (especially IgM).

2. Spleen opsonizes foreign material to enhance recognition by B-cells, especially important in encapsulated bacteria, i.e., pneumococcus, meningococcus, hemophilus.

III. Splenic removal

A. Non-trauma

1. Splenic removal may be needed because of:

   (a) abnormal function (i.e. ITP (idiopathic thrombocytopenic purpura) in which the spleen makes abnormal antibodies to platelets or other blood elements (remove spleen if patient unresponsive to steroids), or

   (b) normal splenic function with abnormal stresses (i.e., hereditary spherocytosis, thalassemias, etc. - normal splenic function on abnormal RBCs leaves the patient anemic), or

   (c) involvement in or diagnosis of malignant diseases (i.e., staging lap for Hodgkin's lymphoma, etc.).

B. Trauma

1. Tears of the splenic capsule can occasionally be followed with serial CT scans or U/S to try to salvage the spleen.

2. Deeper lacerations may be repaired with sutures or compressive nets.

3. Severe splenic injuries, especially when associated with other life-threatening injuries, are treated with splenectomy.

C. Consequences of removal

1. Primary concern is lack of opsonization of encapsulated bacteria, esp. Strep

pneumococcus, leading to overwhelming sepsis and death.

2. Incidence of this complication is very low in trauma patients (1-2% in adults) and still fairly low in patients having splenectomy for hematologic reasons (approx 5%).

3. Give pneumococcal vaccine preoperatively when possible, but certainly postoperatively.

4. Children may benefit from penicillin prophylaxis as in rheumatic fever.

IV. Other

A. Splenic cysts or abscesses can occur but are unusual and usually are treated with splenectomy.

GASTROINTESTINAL HEMORRHAGE

I. **Upper GI bleeding**

   A. General approach

      1. Obtain history and physical exam

      2. Begin IV hydration with large bore peripheral IV's.

      3. Monitor adequacy of hydration by blood pressure, heart rate, mental function and urinary output.

      4. Begin efforts to stop bleeding and clearing clots with lavage of the stomach with room temperature water.

      5. Early endoscopy is helpful to identify the bleeding site and many times is helpful to stop bleeding with injection sclerotherapy.

      6. IV Pitressin resulting in splanchnic arterial constriction greatly reduces upper GI bleeding from esophageal varices, gastritis and even peptic ulcer disease.

      7. Patients bleeding from gastric esophageal varices may be controlled with the use of gastric and esophageal balloons (Sengstaken-Blakemore tube).

      8. It is important to correct clotting factors and fluid and electrolyte abnormalities in preparation for possible surgical intervention.

   B. Etiologies of UGI hemorrhage

      1. The most common cause in non-alcoholic patients is peptic ulcer disease.

a. Posterior, duodenal and pyloric channel ulcers which erode into the gastroduodenal artery are most commonly the cause.

b. When a visible vessel is identifiable on endoscopy, chance of recurrent bleeding is extremely high.

2. Gastritis - common etiology of bleeding in alcoholics and non-alcoholics.

a. May result from diffuse gastric wall irritation from external agents (ASA, ETOH, steroids, NSAIDS, etc.) or from ischemic deterioration of the gastric wall from within.

b. Treatment consists of antacids, H_2 blockers, general supportive measures of the patient and correction of clotting factors.

c. Total gastrectomy may be necessary if these measures do not control the bleeding.

3. Esophageal varices - common etiology in alcoholics along with gastritis.

a. Approximately one-third of the patients with esophageal varices will at some time bleed.

b. Of patients who bleed, 75% will re-bleed within one year and 60% will die from bleeding complications within one year.

c. Acute management in addition to the above measures, includes endoscopy with injection sclerotherapy which stops the hemorrhage in approximately 90%.

d. Definitive management of the esophageal varices usually involves operative intervention since injection sclerotherapy is complicated by esophageal ulcers and the development of gastric varices, which cannot be sclerosed.

e. Surgical options for the management of varices include non-selective portal systemic shunts (portacaval shunts and mesocaval shunts, which have a re-bleeding rate of approximately 5-10% and an associated encephalopathy rate 20-30%) and selective variceal decompression procedures (distal splenorenal shunt, which has a re-bleeding rate of 5-10% and an encephalopathy rate of 5-10%). Definitive management of these patients may involve hepatic transplantation in patients who meet the other criteria for liver transplants.

4.   Mallory-Weiss syndrome

    a.   Linear tear at the esophageal junction associated with severe hard episodes of emesis.

    b.   Usually self-limited with correction of the etiology of emesis, generally will resolve.

C.   Indications for operation

1.   Exsanguinating hemorrhage with hypotension upon admission to the hospital.

2.   Loss of greater than six units of blood in the first 12 hours in the hospital.

3.   Re-bleeding in the hospital after 24 hours of cessation of hemorrhage.

4.   Presence of a visible vessel in the bed of the bleeding ulcer site.

II.   **Lower GI bleeding**

A.   General approach

1.   Resuscitative efforts and coagulation defect corrections as indicated in I.A. above is indicated.

2.   Diagnostic efforts for patients presenting with hematochezia should rely heavily on arteriography to localize the site of bleeding.

3.   Tagged RBC studies to localize site of bleeding can be helpful for amounts less than 2 cc's per minute. Arteriography requires 3-4 cc's per minute to identify the bleeding site.

4.   Presence of melena may occur with sources of GI blood loss anywhere from the oral pharynx to the rectum and simply indicates presence of blood within the GI tract for more than a few hours.

    a.   Investigation of melena should begin with the upper GI tract, since it is more common.

B.   Etiology

1. Massive GI bleeding - most commonly due to diverticulosis of the colon.

2. Telangiectasias (AV malformations) of the colonic wall are also a common cause of significant lower GI bleeding.

3. Ulcerative colitis, cancer of the colon, colonic polyps and other various etiologies are less common sources of lower GI bleeding.

C. Management

1. Lower GI bleeding can be localized with arteriography or other localization studies, which continue to bleed in spite of correction of coagulation defects should be treated with operative removal of the offending area.

2. Operative exploration of lower GI bleeding without identifiable source is rarely useful in identifying the source.

III. **GI hemorrhage in infants and children**

A. Upper GI bleed in infants and children is most commonly from esophageal varices due to prehepatic occlusion of the portal vein.

1. Usually self-limited and can be treated with fluid resuscitation and injection sclerotherapy.

B. Intussusception resulting in bright red blood in the stool of an infant around the age of 2 is the most common cause of lower GI bleeding in young children.

a. Meckel's diverticulum with ectopic mucosa may also be the source of bleeding in young children.

HERNIAS

I. Groin hernias

A. Indirect hernia

1. These result from a persistent patent processus vaginalis and thus are considered congenital in origin, although they may not become manifest until later in life.

2. Hernia contents descend through the internal ring lateral to the inferior epigastric vessels, descend down the spermatic cord toward and sometimes into the scrotum.

3. The most common type of hernia in any age or sex group.

4. Development in elderly ages may be associated with COPD and chronic cough, straining on urination due to prostatic disease, straining on defecation due to colonic disease (including colon cancers), etc.

5. Treated by reduction of the hernia mass, closure of the internal ring and in adults is usually associated with repair of the floor of the inguinal canal (Bassini repair or McVay repair).

6. Recurrence rate with first time repair is 2.5-5%, this increases with each subsequent repair.

B. Direct hernia

1. Associated with defect in the fascia of the floor of the inguinal canal - Hesselbach's triangle bounded by the rectus sheath medially and superiorly, inguinal ligament inferiorly and the inferior epigastric vessels laterally.

2.   Less commonly associated with incarceration or strangulation.

3.   Associated with chronic use and significant strain on muscle and fascia layers, including COPD, BPH and colon cancer.

4.   Repair usually involves tight closure of the internal ring and repair of the floor of the canal by Bassini method or McVay repair.

C.   Femoral hernia

1.   Herniation of the intra-abdominal contents through the femoral canal bounded laterally by the femoral vein, anteriorly by the inguinal ligament, posteriorly by the rim of the pubis.

2.   More common in women than in men.

3.   Felt to have an increased incidence of incarceration or strangulation.

4.   Repair requires suprainguinal ligament repair of the McVay type.

D.   Complications

1.   Incarceration - indicates inability of the hernia contents to be reduced to their normal position.

2.   Strangulation - indicates occlusion of the vascular supply to the hernia contents and results in much greater morbidity and mortality.

3.   Sliding hernia in which part of the wall of the hernia is an intra-abdominal content, on the right side this is most commonly cecum and the left side may be bladder wall or sigmoid. In young females, this commonly involves the ovaries.

4.   Richter's hernia involves incarceration of partial wall of bowel in the hernia opening, may lead to necrosis of the bowel wall without signs of intestinal obstruction.

II.   Other hernia

A.   Umbilical hernias

1.   Most common in young children and often resolve by the age of two when the patient begins to walk. Large umbilical hernias or those occurring in

adults may be repaired with a few simple sutures to prevent incarceration and strangulation.

B.   Incisional hernia

    1.   These hernias occur after previous operative procedures, usually from the result of wound infection, necrosis of the fascia, breakage of sutures or other technical problems.

    2.   May be associated with incarceration or strangulation.

    3.   Repair is usually indicated and must involve getting back to normal, healthy fascia.

C.   Ventral hernia

    1.   Ventral hernias involve those of the abdominal wall (other than incisional hernias). Umbilical hernias are a special type of ventral hernia.

    2.   Other special types of ventral hernia, include Spigelian hernia (herniation at the semilunar line of the rectus sheath and the semicircular line of Douglas) and Petit's triangle hernia (herniation through the inferior lumbar triangle posteriorly).

    3.   These hernias may incarcerate or strangulate and usually do require repair with reapproximation of normal fascial boundaries.

BREAST

I. Anatomy/Physiology

A. Anatomic changes parallel physiologic changes especially in female breast.

B. Breast is a subcutaneous apocrine gland with a blood supply from the chest wall vessels (intercostals, internal mammary, etc.) and a lymphatic system which follows this same pathway - most importantly draining into the axilla.

C. Histologic structure consists of adipose tissue with lobules (12-24) of mammary glands which connect through ducts, ultimately emptying into multiple ducts in the nipple.

D. Stromal elements and fibrous tissue predominate in the young female, giving way to more glands and ducts during the reproductive years (esp. during pregnancy and lactation) and finally becoming more fatty tissue as the ducts and glands involute after menopause. Similar changes occur, to a lesser extent, during menstrual periods under the influence of varying hormonal changes.

E. During lactation, milk is actively expressed from the nipple by myointimal cells.

II. Evaluation

A. Physical exam by the patient is recommended at monthly intervals and by a physician at yearly intervals.

B. Mammography recommendations include baseline exam between 35-40 years; every other year exam, ages 40-50; yearly exam after 50 years old. Patients with high risk factors for development of breast cancer may benefit from more frequent exams.

C.   Ominous characteristics on mammography include clusters of microcalcifications, asymmetric densities, especially those with radiating arms, and skin and nipple retraction.

D.   Stromal tissue in women < 30 years old renders interpretation of mammograms virtually impossible.

E.   Xeromammography is less accurate but can be useful.

F.   Thermography has not been reliable.

III.   Benign conditions

A.   Fibroadenomas

    1.   Benign fibrous nodules, more common in younger women, that are often tender and vary with estrogen flux - usually are well circumscribed. Local excision recommended for symptomatic lesions or difficulty in distinguishing from cancer.

B.   Fibrocystic disease

    1.   Benign process of cyst formation, more common as women get older, present to some extent in most women.

    2.   Present as tender nodules which change during the menstrual cycle.

    3.   Diagnosis with ultrasound or needle aspiration is often sufficient.

    4.   Symptomatic lesions, those that recur after aspiration, or those that have a residual mass after aspiration should be excised.

    5.   Cysts and fibroadenomas appear similar on mammography.

C.   Foci of cellular atypia

    1.   May occur with biopsy of any mass lesion and incidence varies with how diligently it is sought.

    2.   Greater degrees of atypia suggest greater chances of malignancies.

D.   Other

1. Includes fat necrosis, breast abscess, cystosarcoma phylloides, lipoma, papilloma, etc.

IV. Malignant conditions

A. General

1. One out of ten women will develop breast cancer during her life.

2. Breast cancer is the leading cause of cancer deaths of women in United States.

3. Risk factors leading to an increased incidence of breast cancer include:

   a. previous cancer in the opposite or same breast

   b. close blood relative (mother or sister) with breast cancer

   c. early menarche/late menopause

   d. late first pregnancy

   e. nulliparity

B. Ductal carcinoma

1. Most common form - subcategories include:

   a. carcinoma in situ or lobular

   b. comedo

   c. Paget's disease

   d. medullary

   e. colloid or mucinous

   f. tubular

   g. scirrhous (infiltrating ductal)

   h. inflammatory carcinoma

2. Diagnosis

    a. Physical exam - firm, non-tender mass, fixed to underlying tissues, peau d'orange, nipple retraction, axillary nodes.

    b. Mammography - asymmetric density with radiating arms; microcalcifications.

    c. Biopsy of the lesion.

3. Clinical staging

    a. Tumor < 2 cm, no nodes, no distant metastasis - Stage I

    b. Tumor < 2 cm, + nodes, no distant metastasis - Stage II

    c. Tumor > 2 cm, + node, no distant metastasis - Stage III

    d. Tumor > 2 cm, + node, + distant metastasis - Stage IV

    e. Axillary node involvement can often not be accurately assessed from exam only.

4. Treatment

    a. For Stage I and some Stage II lesions, segmentectomy with axillary node dissection, usually followed by chest wall radiation (to prevent a 15-20% local recurrence rate) may be offered.

    b. Most common procedure in United States is modified radical mastectomy - removes whole breast plus axillary contents and is not usually followed with radiation.

    c. Tumors involving chest wall muscles may require a classic radical mastectomy which also removes pectoralis major and minor muscles.

    d. Adjunctive treatment

        (1) Tissue is tested for estrogen (ER) and progesterone (PR) receptors. Pre-menopausal women with ER +, PR + tumors seem to benefit from anti-estrogen therapy.

        (2) Patients with nodal or other distant metastasis benefit from

additional chemotherapy - usually using 3 drugs.

    (3)   Radiation therapy is usually reserved for bony metastasis or inflammatory carcinomas.

    e.   Carcinoma in situ has become much more frequently diagnosed due to improved mammographic techniques and is generally treated by wide local excision, although some authors advocate full cancer operations.

5.   Survival results

    a.   nodes negative - 10 year survival - 72-76%

    b.   nodes positive (overall) - 10 year survival - 25-48%

    c.   1-3 nodes - 10 year survival - 34-68%

    d.   24 nodes - 10 year survival - 14-27%

    e.   metastatic disease - 10 year survival - 0

C.   Lobular carcinoma

1.   Much more rare than ductal carcinoma.

2.   Lobular carcinoma-in-situ is most frequently found as an incidental finding during biopsy of some other lesion and has an approximately 25% incidence of bilaterality.

3.   Natural history is slow and variable but thought to be an indication of increased cancer risk to the patient over time.

4.   Classic treatment meant simple mastectomy plus biopsy of the opposite side. Most are currently treated with wide local excision and close observation.

5.   Invasive lobular carcinomas are generally treated similarly to ductal carcinomas.

VASCULAR SYSTEM

I. **Atherosclerotic peripheral arterial disease**

    A.   Occlusive arterial disease

        1.   Development of atherosclerosis (AS) begins with development of "fatty streaks" in intima and over time develops into a cholesterol plaque involving intima and inner one half of media.

            a.   Deposition of lipids in arterial wall may be response to injury, platelet-endothelium interaction, low or varying wall shear stress and turbulence.

            b.   Risk factors for development of AS include genetic predisposition, diet high in cholesterol and triglycerides, (diet high in animal fats), tobacco use, high blood pressure, high blood sugar, sedentary life style, male sex, and others.

            c.   Risk factor reduction, especially control of high blood pressure, reduction of serum lipids (LDL) and cessation of tobacco have proven to slow or reverse progression of AS.

        2.   Acute arterial occlusion

            a.   Results from emboli lodging at arterial bifurcations (common femoral, popliteal or aortic) or distally (source of emboli = heart or higher in arterial tree, AS plaque or aneurysm) or from acute thrombosis of a chronically diseased artery. Trauma to an artery may also cause acute occlusion.

            b.   Symptoms include acute onset of pain, decreased pulses, pallor, paresthesias with numbness, eventually paralysis and coolness (polar). In a previously normal extremity, irreversible neuro-muscular injury will occur in approximately 6 hours.

c.   In patients with embolic occlusion of previously normal arteries, symptoms and examination are usually all that is necessary for diagnosis. Doppler ultrasound is occasionally helpful - arteriography is time-consuming and not usually necessary.

  (1)   Treatment consists of initial heparinization to prevent propagation of clot and then opening the artery (usually the common femoral) to remove all of the clot with a balloon tipped catheter.

  (2)   Thrombolytic agents have been used successfully when given intra-arterially to patients with very distal emboli unreachable with a catheter.

  (3)   The source of the embolus must be sought and treated.

d.   Acute thrombotic occlusion of diseased arteries often requires arteriography to plan reconstruction.

  (1)   Occurs in the setting of a patient with diffuse PVD who suffers an acute MI with low cardiac output resulting in thrombosis of a peripheral artery or an elderly patient who becomes dehydrated after a bout with the flu, etc.

  (2)   Intra-arterial thrombolytic agents and operative intervention are used when heparin alone is insufficient, depending on the condition of the patient and the extremity.

3.   Chronic arterial occlusive disease

a.   Patients present with 1) exercise induced pain, aching or fatigue in a muscle group distal to the obstructing lesion (intermittent claudication), 2) pain, even at rest in the distal distribution of the arterial system involved - usually the toes or feet - in addition to this, erythematous skin with edema and loss of hair (rest pain) or 3) ulcers or sores which will not heal in spite of adequate local care.

b.   Most commonly involved areas are the aorto-iliac segment (LeRiche syndrome), the distal SFA (at Hunter's canal or the adductor canal), and third, the tibioperoneal arteries.

c.   Diagnosis of the physiologic consequences of arterial occlusion is by non-invasive vascular testing of flow velocities and turbulence as measured by Doppler ultrasound and blood pressures in the leg and ankle compared to the arm (ankle:arm index). Other NIVL tests include pulse volume recording, transcutaneous PO_2 levels and Duplex ultrasound visualization of the arteries.

d.   66% of patients with claudication improve or remain stable with treatment of 1) discontinue tobacco, 2) risk factor reduction, especially initiating a walking exercise program, 3) good foot hygiene. Some patients benefit from reduction of blood viscosity or agents to change RBC deformability (pentoxifylline). Vasodilators or antispasmodics have not been helpful. Only 5% come to major amputation in five years.

e.   33% of patients worsen or wish to have an intervention because of an intolerable lifestyle.

(1)   Short segment stenoses or occlusions of the iliac and femoral systems do well with percutaneous balloon angioplasty (PTA) - 60 to 70%, 3 year patency rates. Intra-arterial stents may be useful in some areas to maintain patency.

(2)   Long segment occlusions of aorto-iliac segments are usually replaced by an aorto-bifemoral bypass graft, perioperative mortality approximately 4%; 85% - 10 year patency.

(3)   SFA occlusive lesions not amenable to PTA may be treated with femoral-popliteal bypass using saphenous vein (60%, 5 year patency) or prosthetic (40-50%, 5 year patency).

(4)   Popliteal and tibioperoneal disease may be treated with vein bypass as far down as the plantar arch vessels - 5 year patency, approximately 60%.

(5)   Longterm careful follow-up with secondary intervention is important for long term limb salvage.

4.   Diabetes mellitus

a.   Patients with diabetes develop histologically routine AS at an earlier age, in a more diffuse form, involving more distal arteries than their non-diabetic counterparts.

b. Early calcification in the walls of the arteries make the usefulness of blood pressure assessments in the lower extremities less useful.

c. Severe tibioperoneal artery involvement is very common.

d. Diabetic neuropathy leading to inadvertent injury and often slow recognition of the injury by the patient, poor leukocyte function and poor arterial perfusion all lead to common foot problems and wound healing problems in patients with diabetes.

e. PTA and bypass grafts with suitable conduits can be as efficacious in patients with diabetes mellitus as those without.

B. Extra-cranial cerebrovascular disease

1. Emboli of atherosclerotic debris from disease at the carotid bifurcation is thought to play a role in approximately 75% of strokes.

2. Symptoms other than stroke include TIA's (transient ischemic attacks - focal neurologic deficits which resolve completely < 24 hours), amaurosis fugax (transient monocular blindness due to Hollenhorst plaque - AS emboli in ophthalmic artery) and RIND (reversible ischemic neurologic deficit resolving < 7 days).

3. Patients usually have bruit in neck (but may not and presence or absence of bruit does not correlate with degree of stenosis) and stigmata of AS disease in other organ systems - especially the heart.

4. Diagnostic evaluation includes Duplex U/S to assess the degree of stenosis and the morphology of the plaque and/or OPG (oculopneumoplethys-mography) to indirectly gauge the degree of stenosis. CT scan or MR scan often reveal previous undetected cerebral scars.

5. Arteriography is usually done prior to operation to look for AS disease in sites other than the carotid bifurcation (aortic arch, intracranial, etc.)

6. Risk of stroke in a patient with TIAs is 5-6%/year and two recent studies have shown superior patient outcome when symptomatic patients with > 75% stenosis are treated with carotid endarterectomy. Expected perioperative stroke rate 2-4%, mortality 1-2%.

7.   Asymptomatic patient with critical stenoses (> 90%) may do better with endarterectomy versus ASA alone if perioperative stroke rate is < 2%.

8.   Recurrent symptomatic rate after CEA is approximately 1%/year (similar to population) but restenosis rate may be 10-15%.

9.   Bilateral carotid disease along with bilateral vertebral artery disease may lead to "vertebrobasilar symptoms" of paraplegia, dizziness plus speech or hemiplegia problems, bilateral blindness episodes, etc. and may be improved by carotid endarterectomy (or occasionally repair/revision of vertebral artery).

10. Subclavian steal syndrome is the onset of vertebrobasilar symptoms with exercise of left arm, due to occlusion of left subclavian artery proximal to vertebral artery, resulting in reversal of flow in the vertebral to supply the arm. Symptoms improve with carotid-subclavian bypass or PTA of subclavian artery. If patient has no symptoms, nothing is done.

C.   Aneurysms

1.   Thoracic aortic aneurysms

   a.   Three major types of AS aneurysms (ascending, arch and descending) - can also be caused by infection (syphilis) or cystic medial necrosis (Marfan syndrome).

      (1)   Ascending and descending are relatively easily repaired with grafts but arch aneurysms cause problems with perfusion to brain etc.

   b.   Traumatic aneurysms due to blunt trauma occur at or just distal to ligamentum arteriosum and are "false"aneurysms (having no true arterial wall) needing graft replacement.

   c.   Dissecting aneurysms are related to hypertension as well as AS and present as sudden, tearing chest pain.

      (1)   DeBakey Type I, II, III - depending on site of entry and exit points.

      (2)   Diagnosis made with CT scan and/or arteriography.

      (3)   Repair concentrates on repair of point of initiation of the

dissection plus ensuring adequate flow to end organs.

2. Abdominal aortic aneurysm (AAA)

    a. Most common aneurysm found - 95% below renal artery.

    b. Associated with AS but also has a degenerative component to its development that may be genetic (anti-thrombin III deficiency, increased elastase activity, etc.)

    c. Natural history is that of a variable rate of enlargement (with more rapid rates occurring as the aneurysm enlarges) and leakage/rupture at varying sizes (although rupture rate increases as size increases).

    d. Other complications include distal embolization of clot or AS plaque and local compression of surrounding organs.

    e. U/S is useful for size measurement, but CT also good and reveals more information regarding neck of aneurysm and concomitant disease.

    f. Arteriography helpful to plan reconstruction if patient is a claudicator or to look for renal involvement if patient is hypertensive.

    g. Aneurysms over 5 cm should be repaired as the risk of rupture (30% in 3 years) is greater than the risk of dying from other causes. Aneurysm 4-5 cm should be repaired if the patient is in good health - can be followed by ultrasound to observe for evidence of enlargement if patient is not a good operative candidate.

    h. Repair usually means replacement of the involved segment of artery with graft material. Operative mortality is 2-4%. Induced thrombosis of the aneurysm with extra-anatomic bypass can be useful in high risk patients.

3. Peripheral aneurysms

    a. Other common sites include the common femoral arteries and popliteal arteries.

    b. High incidence of bilateral aneurysms (25%) and 50% are associated with AAA.

c. Repair indicated at any size to prevent the complications of 1) acute thrombosis or 2) distal embolization. (Rupture can occur but is unusual).

d. Other intra-abdominal aneurysms include those involving the splenic, renal or hepatic arteries or any other artery in the abdomen (in decreasing frequency). All are mostly associated with AS and most have a low incidence of rupture especially if the wall has calcified.

D. Non-atherosclerotic arterial disease.

1. Raynaud's syndrome - a vasospastic disorder, more common in women than men, of unknown etiology, manifested by abnormally severe reaction of fingers and hands to cold exposure. Usually a benign condition treated with gloves or low-dose vasodilating agents, i.e., calcium channel blockers. May be associated with other autoimmune disorders, i.e., SLE, anticardiolipin antibody syndrome, scleroderma, rheumatoid arthritis, etc.

2. Buerger's disease - arteritis obliterans - a disease of smokers, men > women, involving progressive obliteration of small and medium sized arteries of the hands and feet. Commonly leads to amputations. Treatment involves complete abstinence from tobacco.

3. Polyarteritis nodosa - autoimmune complex disease that can lead to microaneurysm formation or obliterative processes in the small vessels.

II. Venous Disease

A. Deep vein thrombosis (DVT)

1. Etiology - Virchow's triad: stasis, vessel injury, hypercoagulable state.

2. High risk groups for development include females, elderly, overweight, immobile, cancer, previous history of DVT, orthopedic procedures, etc.

3. Preventive measures include low dose heparin (5000 U SQ q 12 hours), calf pumps, early ambulation. For orthopedic patients, dextran or full anticoagulation.

4. Diagnosis - clinical signs/symptoms of painful, swollen calf with + Homan's sign is only approximately 50 percent accurate.

a. Non-invasive tests include duplex ultrasound, impedance plethysmography, and venous Doppler exam.

b. Venography is the radiographic choice.

5. Treatment is anticoagulation for 6 - 12 weeks, first with heparin, then with warfarin.

6. Thrombolytic agents dissolve clots faster but are more expensive and ultimate value are still in question.

7. Complications of DVT include pulmonary emboli (PE) and venous valvular insufficiency (post-phlebitic syndrome).

B. Pulmonary embolism

1. Common cause or contributing factor to deaths in the hospital.

2. Manifestations include sudden chest pain, SOB, tachypnea, feeling of impending doom, hypoxia, occasionally hemoptysis. These are often absent.

3. Diagnosis most reliably made with pulmonary angiogram. Nuclear lung scans are used commonly and can be helpful along with chest x-ray and compatible clinical scenario.

4. Treatment usually involves 3 - 6 months anticoagulation (heparin followed by warfarin) but thrombolytics may have value in lysing clots faster and more thoroughly, leading to less long-term pulmonary arterial resistance.

5. Patients with recurrent PE on anticoagulation, complications to anticoagulants or contraindication to anticoagulation should be protected with an IVC filter (Greenfield or "Bird's nest" filters are most commonly used).

C. Venous valvular insufficiency

1. Causes include malformed valves, chronic stress leading to valve failure, and injury to the valve after thrombosis.

2. Superficial valvular incompetence leads to varicose veins which can be treated with graded elastic support hose or, if symptoms such as phlebitis, bleeding or severe cosmetic deformity result, can be excised (stripping) or

sometimes treated with injection sclerotherapy.

3.   Incompetence of the perforating veins and/or deep vein valves leads to swelling, pigmentation of the skin, symptoms of heaviness, aching, etc, and occasionally ulcers in the "gaiter" area of the medial and lateral malleolus. Treatment consists of elevation and external support with stockings as well as local wound care.

III.   Lymphatic disorders

A.   Lymphedema of unknown etiology occurring before age 35 years is lymphedema praecox, generally due to congenitally small lymphatics and most often becomes manifested in second or third decade of life.

B.   Lymphedema at birth is Milroy's disease.

C.   Lymphedema occurring after age 35 is lymphedema tarda and usually occurs because of obliteration of lymphatics which were probably small originally.

D.   Secondary lymphedema occurs following destruction of major lymph draining areas by surgery, trauma, cancer, infection or radiation - most commonly involves groin to leg or axilla to arm.

    1.   Long-standing acquired lymphedema may predispose to lymphosarcoma.

E.   Treatment is primarily elevation, graded elastic support hose and careful treatment of injuries to prevent cellulitis and lymphangitis.

    1.   Graded mechanical pumping can reduce the swelling as well.

    2.   Reduction surgery to get rid of excess tissue (occasionally) is useful.

F.   On rare occasions, normal lymph vessels will drain into an area that becomes obstructed, leading to dilated lymph channels. These can sometimes be anastomosed to normal veins to promote lymphatic drainage.

HEART

I. Congenital disease

A. Left to right shunt

1. Patent ductus arteriosus (PDA)

    a. Normal closure occurs in a full term neonate within the first 10-15 hours mediated by lower levels of Prostaglandin E series - complete closure is complete in 88% of newborns by 8 weeks.

    b. Prolonged patency results in a left to right shift with pulmonary congestion and left ventricular volume overload.

    c. Incidence increases with prematurity and decrease in birth weight.

    d. Manifested by a hyperdynamic cardiac function and continuous "machinery"murmur.

    e. Usually managed by transthoracic ligation - can occasionally be managed by transcatheter occlusion with "Ivalon"plug.

2. Atrial septal defect (ASD)

    a. The fifth most common congenital cardiac abnormality with no known precise etiology. Increased incidence with trisomy 21, Marfan syndrome and Turner's syndrome.

    b. Ostium secundum defects are the most common with ostium primum defects and arterial ventricular canal defects being more severe degrees and similar hemodynamic abnormalities.

c. With increasing degrees of defects, there is increasing degree of left to right shunt with pulmonary hypertension resulting from the increased pulmonary flow.

d. These lesions become manifest relatively early, depending on the degree of shunting. Treatment is either primary or patch closure of the defect.

3. Total anomalous pulmonary venous return

a. All of the oxygenated pulmonary venous blood mixes with desaturated systemic blood in the right atrium.

b. Right atrial output reaches the systemic circulation through persistent ASD, VSD or PDA.

c. There are at least four different subtypes of TAPVR.

d. Infants without pulmonary venous obstruction are usually tachypneic at birth but may not appear cyanotic.

e. Congestive heart failure becomes progressively worse without surgical therapy, 75% will die before one year of age.

f. Operative correction requires anastomosis of the common pulmonary venous channel to the left atrium and obliteration of the anomalous venous connection. Operative mortality in infants is decreased to approximately 25% with good prognosis for those who survive.

4. Ventricular septal defects (VSD)

a. Isolated VSD is the most common congenital cardiac anomaly, accounting for 30-40% of all congenital lesions at birth.

b. Four general anatomic types are: supracristal or subarterial VSD, high or perimembranous VSD, arterial ventricular canal type defects, muscular type defects.

c. The direction and magnitude of shunt depends upon the size of the defect and difference in pressure between the ventricles in systole and diastole. When the defect is large, it offers little resistance to flow and relatively small pressure differences may result in significant flow across the defect. Early repair of large defects is generally indicated to prevent the development of pulmonary artery hypertension.

B.   Right to left shunt

1.   Tetralogy of Fallot (TOF)

   a.   One of the most frequent serious cardiac conditions accompanied by cyanosis in which infants develop symptoms within the first six weeks of life.

   b.   There are a number of variations and anatomic changes in this disease. Dextro position of the aorta and hypertrophy of the right ventricle, along with pulmonary stenosis and VSD are the four primary anatomic defects.

   c.   The two most important malformations are obstruction of the right ventricular outflow tract and the ventricular septal defect (resulting in right to left shunt).

   d.   Most patients with TOF are candidates for operative repair, preferably between the ages of 3 and 5, except in the more severe forms which require early operative intervention.

   e.   Subclavian to pulmonary artery anastomosis (Blalock-Taussig) is an excellent operation in patients who are not a suitable candidate for total correction.

   f.   The corrective procedure can be done with a mortality of approximately 5% . This is complicated by occurrence of heart block during closure of the VSD or congestive heart failure due to failing right ventricle.

2.   Transposition of the great vessels (TGV)

   a.   With complete transposition, the aorta rises anteriorly from the anatomic right ventricle and the pulmonary artery rises from the anatomic left ventricle.

   b.   Associated anomalies which permit life include patent ductus arteriosus, patent foramen of ovale, VSD and left ventricular outflow tract obstruction.

c. Transposition is the leading cause of death resulting from congenital heart disease in early life. The patient presents in the first week of life with cyanosis. If they have inadequate mixing, this can be improved by creating an atrial septal defect (Rashkind procedure).

d. The Mustard operation switches the great arteries plus coronary arteries for complete repair. Senning employed a technique to create the first intra-atrial repair. Jatene has also reported success in switching the great arteries with reimplantation of the coronary arteries.

II. Acquired cardiac disease

A. Coronary artery disease (CAD)

1. CAD is the most common cause of death in the Western world and is thought to be the result of a combination of genetic predisposition, atherogenic diet, hypertension, sedentary lifestyle, tobacco abuse and diabetes.

2. Manifested by angina pectoris (exercise induced chest pain) or acute myocardial infarction with acute occlusion to coronary artery circulation.

3. Most patients with chronic, stable myocardial ischemia can be managed by appropriate pharmacologic therapy, including nitroglycerin, beta blockers and calcium antagonists.

4. Transarterial balloon dilatation (PTCA) of proximal lesions in the coronary arteries can be done safely to improve perfusion of the myocardial wall.

5. In general, revascularization is recommended for patients with double and triple coronary artery disease, including all of those with left main coronary artery lesions. Coronary artery bypass grafting increases longevity as well as providing distinct symptomatic improvement.

   a. Patients with unstable angina not responsive to pharmacologic agents are also suitable for balloon angioplasty or bypass grafting.

6. Mortality and morbidity

   a. Perioperative death rate should be under 10%.

   b. Complete relief of pain occurs in more than two-thirds of all patients.

    c.   Improved left ventricular function has been shown following successful bypass.

    d.   Patency rate of bypass grafts is approximately 86% at one year.

    e.   Saphenous vein patency at ten years is recently noted to be 53%, whereas internal mammary artery patency in the same series is 84%.

B.   Acquired aortic valve disease

    1.   Rheumatic aortic stenosis due to rheumatic fever secondary to Group A Streptococci infection and calcific aortic stenosis occurring primarily in congenital bicuspid valves are the most common sources for aortic stenosis.

    2.   Significant aortic stenosis results in clinical manifestation of chest pain, syncope, and congestive failure.

        a.   Effort syncope has been related to arrhythmias and may lead to sudden death syndrome.

    3.   Patients with significant symptoms of aortic stenosis have a poor, long-term prognosis and are, in general, candidates for operative correction.

    4.   Aortic valve insufficiency

        a.   Intrinsic diseases of the valve, particularly rheumatic fever, bacterial endocarditis or congenital bicuspid valves may lead to aortic insufficiency.

        b.   Cystic medial necrosis or intimal tears in the lining of the ascending aorta may result in stretching of the aortic valve ring and valvular insufficiency.

        c.   The common manifestations are that of rising left ventricular filling pressures and symptoms of congestive failure - dyspnea, fatigue, orthopnea, paroxysmal nocturnal dyspnea.

        d.   Patients with symptomatic insufficiency are candidates for valve replacement which is the operation of choice.

    5.   The overall operative mortality rate for aortic valve replacement is

approximately 7%.

C.   Acquired mitral valve disease

    1.   Mitral stenosis (MS)

        a.   Predominant cause is rheumatic fever, although good history for this is present in only one-half of the patients.

        b.   Most patients remain asymptomatic in a latent phase for two decades before the onset of symptoms. Symptoms are those of orthopnea, paroxysmal nocturnal dyspnea, hemoptysis, easy fatigability and episodes of frank pulmonary edema.

        c.   Peripheral cyanosis may be present as well as hepatic enlargement and peripheral edema.

        d.   Surgical approach is indicated when the diagnosis is made because of progressive stenosis of the mitral orifice. Operation is indicated if the mitral orifice size is less than 1 cm per meter square of body surface area.

        e.   Repair consists of either closed or open mitral commissurotomies or mitral valve replacement.

    2.   Mitral regurgitation (MR)

        a.   30-45% of MR requiring operation is from rheumatic valvulitis and is the most common process involving mitral valve.

        b.   The basic pathophysiology is alteration of left atrial blood pressure and left ventricular failure. More important symptoms which develop are dyspnea on exertion, easy fatigability and palpitations.

        c.   Patients with significant MR who begin to develop limitation due to congestive cardiomegaly or pulmonary hypertension should be treated with mitral valve repair or a prosthetic valve replacement.

III.   Pacemakers

A.   The indications for permanent pacing are included in the list below:

    1.   Sick sinus syndrome with bradytachycardia arrhythmia syndrome.

2.   Mobitz Type II AV block

3.   Complete AV block

4.   Symptomatic bilateral bundle branch block

5.   Bivesicular or incomplete trivesicular block with intermittent complete AV block following acute MI.

6.   Carotid sinus syncope

7.   Recurrent drug resistant tachycardia arrhythmias improved by temporary pacing

8.   Intractable low cardiac output syndrome benefitted by temporary pacing

LUNG AND MEDIASTINUM

I.   **Pulmonary functions**

    A.   Most commonly used pulmonary function tests for day to day management of the patients, include:

        1.   Tidal volume (TV) - volume of air inspired during quiet normal respiration.

        2.   Vital capacity (VC) - amount of air that can be expired following maximal inspiration.

        3.   Forced vital capacity (FVC) - volume of air that can be forcibly expired with maximal expiratory effort.

        4.   Forced expiratory volume - one second (FEV_1) - the amount of air that can be forcibly expired in the first second of the FVC.

        5.   Maximum voluntary ventilation (MVV) - the amount of air that can be breathed in one minute during maximum effort calculated for 15 seconds of actual ventilation .

        6. $FEV_1/FVC\%$ - the fraction of the FVC maximum expired in one second

    B.   Numerous other pulmonary function analyses can be made in unusual situations.

    C.   Arterial blood gases - measure the pH of the blood, the partial pressure of oxygen (PaO_2) and carbon dioxide ($PaCO_2$) in arterial blood.

        1.   The pH normally ranges from 7.37 to 7.43 and is maintained by complex - interactions of the blood buffering systems, renal compensation and

ventilatory compensation.

    a.   Acute respiratory alkalosis - low $PaCO_2$ and high pH - common clinical findings resulting from hyperventilation.

    b.   Respiratory acidosis - high $PaCO_2$ and low pH, indicative of hypoventilation.

    c.   Metabolic alkalosis - high pH and low $PaCO_2$, indicative of a metabolic alkalosis.

    d.   Metabolic acidosis, low pH and high $PaCO_2$, indicative of extra acid load.

2.   Oxygen dissociation curve can be used to indicate the effect of temperature and pH on the ability to oxygenate the tissues, as well as demonstrating the rapid decline of PaO_2 that occurs when the oxygen in the blood is lowered from full saturation (O_2 saturation of 90% correlates with a PaO_2 of approximately 60 mmHg).

3. $PaCO_2$ is a direct measure of alveolar ventilation. The normal range is 38-42 mmHg.

C.   Effect of surgical procedures on pulmonary function

1.   The degree of pulmonary dysfunction is directly related to the type of operation and the preoperative status of pulmonary function of the patient.

2.   Total lung capacity is reduced after operations in the upper part of the torso.

3.   Atelectasis results from decreased surface area for gas exchange with collapse of alveoli, resulting in arterial hypoxemia.

4.   Airway closure is due to postoperative splinting of the chest and altered breathing pattern.

D.   Preoperative evaluation of risk

1.   Increased age and smoking history. Increased closing volume.

2.   Obesity diminishes FRC and ERV, resulting in airway closure and atelectasis.

3. An FEV_1 of greater than 2 liters is associated with minimal pulmonary risk after abdominal operations. Increased risks are associated with FEV_1 of 1-2 liters.

4. When FEV_1 is less than 0.8 liters, there is moderate to severe risk of being unable to wean the patient from the ventilator.

II. Lung cancer

A. Risk factors

 1. Cigarette smoking is the primary risk factor in the pathogenesis of carcinoma of the lung in the Western world today.

B. Pathologic types

 1. Squamous cell carcinoma - most common type with incidence of 40-70% of total lesions.

  a. Nearly all of these patients have a cigarette smoking history.

 2. Undifferentiated - in most series represents 20-30% of the total (oatcell lesions).

 3. Adenocarcinoma - occurs in 5-15% and are more often seen peripherally.

  a. Higher incidence in females and higher tendency to metastasize to liver, brain, bone and adrenals, as well as lymph nodes.

 4. Bronchoalveolar carcinoma - very well differentiated neoplasm associated with the most favorable prognosis of pulmonary cancers. The five year survival is 48%.

 5. Giant cell carcinoma - variant of bronchogenic adenocarcinoma, usually aggressive, incidence of 1-10%. Early metastasis.

C. Clinical manifestations

 1. Many patients are asymptomatic at the time of presentation, have an abnormal chest x-ray being done for other reasons.

 2. Among clinical symptoms commonly seen are cough, weight loss, dyspnea, chest pain, hemoptysis, bone pain, clubbing of fingers, presence of superior

vena cava syndrome.

3.   Rare bronchogenic carcinomas produce clinical endocrinopathy, including inappropriate diuresis (ADH secretion), hypercalcemia, carcinoid syndrome and Cushing's syndrome.

4.   Pancoast tumor is one that arises anatomically on the superior sulcus of the lung and can infiltrate the upper mediastinum and brachial plexus and cervical sympathetic nerves.

D.   Establishing a diagnosis

1.   Radioisotope scanning, CT scanning and MRIs can all be used to identify suspected lesions seen on chest x-ray and tomography. These tests also help identify the presence of disease in mediastinal or other lymph nodes.

2.   Biopsy of the lesion either with fine needle aspiration for cytologic studies, through the use of bronchoscopy or through the use of mediastinoscopy to needle aspirate lymph nodes are all important for establishing a diagnosis.

E.   Treatment

1.   With no evidence of metastasis, invasion or obstruction to the thorax, exploratory thoracotomy in an effort to remove the offending lesion is the most commonly successful treatment for most types of lung cancer.

2.   Radiation is frequently employed in a patient with bronchogenic carcinoma and prolongs life by reducing symptoms for those with metastatic lesions in whom resection is inappropriate.

3.   Chemotherapy is particularly useful in patients with small cell carcinoma because of the dismal results with surgery and radiation. Cyclophosphamide with the addition of Vincristine and Doxorubicin (Adriamycin) are particularly helpful.

4.   The natural history of bronchogenic carcinoma is dismal with a one year mortality of 95% if untreated. Patients without known metastasis have five years survival in the 50% range and 30% if only the hilar nodes are positive. Best prognosis is found in patients with solitary peripheral lesions less than 4 cm in diameter.

F.   Solitary "coin" lesion

1.   The younger the patient, the more likely the lesion is to be benign.

2.   Solitary coin lesions are defined as being solitary, round, sharp margins, less than 2 cm in diameter without associated microcalcifications or other associated lesions within the chest.

3.   Evaluation should include review of old chest x-rays, testing for tuberculosis and histoplasmosis and sputum cytology for malignant cells, cultures and tuberculosis. Ultimately bronchoscopy with washings and occasionally a transthoracic needle biopsy may be needed. If no diagnosis can be obtained, thoracotomy and excision of the lesion is indicated.

III.   **Primary tumors and cysts of the mediastinum**

A.   Usual location of mediastinal tumors and cysts:

Anterosuperior	**Middle**	**Posterior**
Thymoma	Lymphoma	Neurogenic tumors
Lymphoma	Carcinoma	Enteric cysts
Germ cell tumors	Pericardial cysts	Bronchogenic cysts
Tetratodermoid	Bronchogenic cysts	Mesenchymal
Malignant germ	Enteric cysts	tumors
cell tumors	Mesenchymal	
Carcinoma	tumors	
Thyroid adenoma		
Parathyroid		
adenoma		
Mesenchymal		
tumors		

1.   Neurogenic tumors are the most common neoplasms encountered in the mediastimum - 21% of all primary tumors and cysts in collected series - are usually located in the posterior mediastimum - 10-20% are malignant.

2.   Thymoma

      a.   Second most frequent lesion in the mediastinum - usually the anterior superior mediastinum

      b.   Peak incidence in third to fifth decade of life.

      c.   May present with symptoms related to local mass effects, including chest pain, dyspnea, hemoptysis, cough or symptoms of superior vena cava obstruction. Thymomas are also frequently associated with myasthenia gravis, occurring in 10-50% of patients with thymomas.

TRANSPLANTATION

I.   General aspects

A.   Definitions

1.   <u>Autograft</u> - tissue transplanted from one site of the body to another in the same individual.

2.   <u>Isograft</u> - tissue transferred between genetically identical individuals (renal transplant between monozygotic twins).

3.   <u>Allograft</u> - tissue transplanted between genetically dissimilar individuals of the same species.

4.   <u>Xenograft</u> - tissue transferred between individuals of a different species.

5.   <u>Orthotopic graft (orthograft)</u> - an organ placed at the normal anatomic position (liver, heart).

6.   <u>Heterotopic graft</u> - organ placed at a site different than a normal anatomic position (as in renal transplantation).

B.   Immunology

1.   Genetic loci for humeral and cellular immune responses are located on the short arm of the sixth chromosome.

2.   Class I antigens are single chain glucoproteins catalogued as HLA, B, or C.

3.   Class I antigens are detected by serologic testing, using lymphocytes and a

known panel of antisera.

    a.   In living related donor kidney transplants, these antigens have a very strong correlation with graft success.

    4.   Class II antigens are glycoproteins, consisting of two polymeric chains containing a common subunit.

        a.   Present on B lymphocytes, dendritic cells, activated T cells, endothelial cells and monocytes.

        b.   Several series within the HLA locus are found including HLA-D and the HLA-D locus.

        c.   These antigens are responsible for the cellular arm of the immune response and are defined by mixed lymphocyte culture test (MLC).

        d.   Because it takes 5-7 days to perform MLC, Class II antigens are generally disregarded except in very elective situations.

C.   Rejection responses

    1.   Hyperacute rejection - occurs minutes to several hours following implantation.

        a.   Associated with preformed antibodies directed toward either ABO blood group or HLA antigens.

        b.   Currently is rare because of cross matching and blood group matching.

    2.   Accelerated acute rejection - occurs during the first several days following transplant.

        a.   In the kidney, is associated with oliguria, DIC, thrombocytopenia and hemolysis.

        b.   Thought to represent a second set of anamnestic responses mediated by both antibodies and lymphocytes.

        c.   Rare type of rejection with no effective treatment.

    3.   Acute rejection - occurs in up to 90 percent of cadaver donor transplants.

a. Characterized by clinical characteristics of organ failure.

b. T-cell infiltration into vascular and interstitial spaces.

c. Treatable with increased doses of immunosuppression and a good prognosis if reversible.

d. Acute rejections may ultimately damage the organ.

4. Chronic rejection - slow progressive immunologic destruction over months to years.

a. Vascular intimal hyperplasia, lymphocytic infiltration, atrophy and fibrosis of renal, cardiac or hepatic tissue.

b. Mediated by humeral and cellular events.

c. Unaltered by increased immunosuppression.

D. Immunosuppressive drug therapy.

1. All immunosuppressive regimens have common side effects of decreased resistance to infection on the part of the host.

a. These infections are frequently opportunistic with Candida, cytomegalovirus, herpes virus and Pneumocystis carinii.

b. Resistance to tumors is also impaired, especially lymphomas and skin cancers.

2. Azathioprine (Imuran) - antimetabolite which inhibits nucleic acid synthesis in all replicating cells of the body.

a. Provides baseline immunosuppression and not used for specific rejection.

b. Frequently used in combination with steroids and Cyclosporin.

c. Has complication of bone marrow depression.

3. Glucocorticosteroids

a. Used in nearly all organ transplants.

b.   Mechanism of action poorly understood but it is lympholytic and inhibits Interleukin I release from macrophages. Commonly used to treat rejection episodes as a pulse therapy, as well as used chronically for baseline immunosuppression.

c.   Complications include development of dyspepsia, cataracts, osteonecrosis of joints, glucose intolerance, acne, capillary fragility and Cushing's syndrome.

4.   Cyclosporin

a.   Blocks the secretion of Interleukin II, a T-cell growth factor; prevents proliferation and maturation of cytotoxic T-cells responsible for graft rejection.

b.   Used for maintenance immunosuppressive therapy in combination with steroids and Azathioprine - has not been helpful for acute cellular rejection.

c.   Complications include dose dependent nephrotoxicity, hypertension, hyperkalemia, hirsutism, gingival hyperplasia, hepatotoxicity, tumors and breast fibroadenomas.

5.   Macrolides - FK506 and Rapamycin

a.   New agents which are fungal metabolites and are potent immunosuppressive agents.

b.   Action seems to be specific for T or B cells.

c.   Act synergistically with steroids and cyclosporin.

6.   Polyclonal antilymphocyte or antithymocyte serums and globulins (ALG, ATG).

a.   Prepared by immunizing an animal with human lymphocytes or thymocytes.

b.   Used to induce immunosuppression immediately after transplant or for the treatment of rejection episodes.

c.   Use of these monoclonal antibodies makes it possible to specifically direct immunosuppressive therapy so that only the cells responsible for rejection episodes, are immunosuppressed.

    d.   OKT$_3$ is the most commonly used such agent.

7.   Other

    a.   <u>Blood transfusion</u>, either donor specific or random donor, has been shown to be productive against rejection - mechanism not well understood.

    b.   <u>Total lymphoid irradiation.</u>

        (1)   Used to prevent occurrence of rejection.

        (2)   Requires pretransplant radiation to all lymph node bearing areas.

    c.   <u>Plasmapheresis</u> is used on highly sensitized recipients as adjunctive therapy for accelerated rejection episode.

    d.   Thoracic duct drainage is used as an outmoded technique, requires cannulation of the thoracic duct with subsequent lymphocyte depletion.

II.   Organ and tissue donation

A.   Criteria for cessation of brain function.

    1.   Absence of spontaneous respirations, plus absence of pupillary light response, plus absence of corneal light reflex, plus absence of oculocephalic or oculovestibular reflex, plus unresponsiveness to stimuli, plus known cause for condition, plus duration of condition over time, plus known irreversibility, suggests brain death!

    2.   Confirmatory tests

        a.   Sustained apnea or disconnecting respiratory.

        b.   EEG

        c.   Radionuclear brain scan

        d.   Cerebral angiography

e.   Confirmatory tests are not mandatory but serve and support the diagnosis of brain death.

B.   Organ acceptability

1.   Acute and chronic diseases affecting certain organs may exclude them for consideration of transplantation.

2.   Helpful lab tests for heart-lung transplants, include cardiac catheterization, echocardiogram, EKG, chest x-ray, CPK enzymes with MB fractionation.

3.   Lab tests for kidney transplants include BUN, creatinine and hypertension check.

4.   For pancreatic transplant - glucose tolerance tests and a careful history are important.

5.   For liver transplant - liver function tests, history of hepatitis B or chronic hepatic disease is important.

6.   All transplant patients receive blood, urine, sputum cultures, hepatitis screening, VDRL and HIV tests.

C.   Organ preservation

1.   Kidney, heart, lung, liver and pancreas are routinely flushed in situ with cold solution to stop metabolism rapidly. They are stored in cold solutions containing electrolytes and osmotic active agents which best maintain cellular preservation.

III.   **Kidney transplantation**

A.   Indication for a kidney transplant is chronic renal failure from any cause, free of other major diseases and between 1 and 70 years of age.

B.   The transplant is nearly always placed as a heterotopic allograft.

C.   Immunosuppression varies from center to center but usually involves the use of Imuran, steroids and cyclosporin, OKT-3 or antithymocyte globulin may be given for acute rejection episodes.

D.   Functional graft survival of 75-85 percent for cadaver kidneys and 95 percent for living related donors at one year is now common. Patient survival of 95 percent at one year is also common.

IV. **Liver transplant**

    A.   Candidates are those with a life expectancy of 1 year or less and free of malignancy or infection.

    B.   Diseases treated with liver transplant include cirrhosis (post necrotic or alcoholic), primary biliary cirrhosis, primary sclerosing cholangitis, metabolic diseases with and without cirrhosis, congenital biliary atresia, congenital hepatic fibrosis.

    C.   Other indications are occasionally indicated as well, including primary liver tumors.

    D.   Transplant is almost always an orthotopic graft from the cadaveric donor.

    E.   Patient and graft survival is approximately 85 percent at one year for patients operated on before the terminal phase of their disease.

V. **Heart, heart-lung and lung transplantation**

    A.   Indication for heart transplant is end stage cardiac failure and the patient is expected to die within six months. Age is not a contraindication. Patient must have full rehabilitation potential.

    B.   Heart-lung transplant is performed where severe pulmonary vascular disease accompanies heart disease.

    C.   The usual heart transplant is an orthotopic allograft that is size matched.

    D.   The current one year graft and patient survival is 80 percent or higher and 5 year rate is 60 to 70 percent.

    E.   Heart-lung transplant recipients can expect 5 year survival rate of 50 percent.

    F.   Single or double lung transplant can provide total pulmonary function to patients with end stage pulmonary disease without suppuration or concomitant cardiac failure.

    G.   Rejection is the most common complication after a lung transplant.

    H.   Results of lung transplant have not been as dramatic as those with heart transplant but are improving with Cyclosporin and steroids.

VI. **Pancreas transplant**

    A.   Indicated in patients with Type I, insulin dependent diabetes and usually concomitant liver failure, vascular disease, retinopathy, neuropathy or enteropathy.

    B.   Most often done with simultaneous renal transplant.

    C.   Many surgical techniques have been used, most commonly transplantation of the entire pancreas with the attached C sweep of the duodenum.

    D.   With routine use of cyclosporin, the one year graft survival of whole organ transplantation is approaching 80 percent.

VII. **Other**

    A.   Allografts of parathyroid tissue, bone and skin have also been successful, as has bone marrow transplantation.

    B.   Small intestine transplant and group organ transplants have been performed but long term success is yet to be achieved.

    C.   Allografts of skin, bone, fascia, dura, endocrine organs, eyes, blood vessels are used clinically in a variety of situations or are being investigated.

ENDOCRINE

I. **Thyroid**

    A. Anatomy

        1. Follicles with supporting stroma and parafollicular cells (C cells).

        2. Right and left lobe plus isthmus which occasionally extends past hyoid bone to foramen cecum at base of tongue.

        3. Arterial supply - inferior thyroid arteries - branches of thyrocervical trunks; superior thyroid arteries are branches of external carotid.

        4. Veins - inferior, middle, superior.

        5. Superior laryngeal nerve runs with superior thyroid artery.

        6. Recurrent laryngeal nerve loops around aortic arch on left, subclavian artery on right, usually travels near tracheoesophageal groove, behind inferior thyroid artery to enter larynx at the inferior cornu of thyroid cartilage.

    B. Physiology

        1. Serum iodine converted to T3 and T4 which have multiple metabolic effects on various end organs (including heart) arteries, fat metabolism, etc.

        2. Parafollicular cells (C cells) secrete calcitonin helps regulate serum calcium level.

    C. The thyroid mass

1. Diagnosis - studies such as thyroid function tests, nuclear scans, ultrasounds or CT/MRI can be done, however, the most useful is needle aspiration with cytologic evaluation.

2. Colloid nodules or "goiters"are most common, are benign, and often resolve with aspiration if cystic. Often in middle aged women.

3. Benign papillary or follicular adenomas may be suggested on needle aspiration but can't be securely diagnosed until the whole nodule is excised.

4. Four common types of primary thyroid cancer histologic types:

   a. Papillary - most common (58%) , tends to be multicentric, relatively rare lymphatic or distant metastasis, treated with lobe plus isthmus resection or total thyroidectomy with 80-90% 10 year survival.

   b. Follicular - second most common, tends to spread to surrounding nodes and distant sites, treated with total thyroidectomy and I-131 for distant metastasis, 60-70% 10 year survival.

   c. Medullary - associated with C cell (Calcitonin production) and MEN II syndrome, commonly recurs or metastasizes, treated with total thyroidectomy, 50% 10 year survival.

   d. Anaplastic - very aggressive tumor with no good treatment alternatives at present, usually treated with debulking procedure to keep tumor off trachea, 0-5 year survivals

5. Other primary and secondary tumors can be found in the thyroid - lymphoma, metastatic cancers, etc.

6. Risk factors associated with higher incidence of cancer include: male gender, young (< 25 year) or old (> 50 yr), history of head and neck radiation, fast growth of mass, hoarseness, tracheal deviation.

D. Hyperthyroidism

1. Hyperfunction of thyroid gland due to a solitary functioning nodule (rare) ("toxic adenoma"), multinodular goiter or diffuse disease (including Grave's disease - most common) is an unusual indication for thyroidectomy.

2. Thyroid "storm"- sudden, massive release of thyroid hormones with hypermetabolic response is also a rare indication for urgent thyroid

operation.

        3.   When possible, control thyroid metabolic activity and end organ response first - propylthiouracil (PTU) and inderal and/or I-131.

        4.   When operation is indicated, total thyroidectomy is usually done.

    E.   Major complications to thyroid operations include injury to recurrent laryngeal nerve (< 1%), permanent hypoparathyroidism (< 1%), other cranial nerve injury (< 2%).

II.   Parathyroid

    A.   Anatomy

        1.   Usually 4 glands - 2 inferior ones derived from 3rd pharyngeal pouch and 2 superior ones from 4th pharyngeal pouch.

        2.   Blood supply from branches of inferior and superior thyroid arteries.

    B.   Physiology

        1.   Produce parathyroid hormone (parathormone)(PTH) in response to a feed back mechanism with serum calcium concentration such that serum calcium concentration is carefully maintained below 8.5 and 10.5 mg/dl. Requires Vitamin D.

    C.   Primary hyperparathyroidism (1° HPT)

        1.   Most common intrinsic cause of hypercalcemia.

            a.   Other causes of hypercalcemia include metastatic cancer to bones, vitamin D/A intoxication, sarcoidosis, multiple myeloma, hyperthyroidism, HCTZ, lithium, milk alkali syndrome.

        2.   Usually diagnosed in an asymptomatic state with persistent elevated serum (Ca^{++}) associated with elevated PTH levels.

        3.   Like hypercalcemia, 1° HPT may be associated with symptoms of peptic ulcer disease, kidney stones, pathologic bone fracture (Brown's tumors), hypertension and psychoses.

        4.   Most common pathology is solitary adenoma.

5. Treated with excision of parathyroid adenoma.

6. Overall most common cause of hypercalcemia is metastatic cancers to bone - especially from lung, breast, colon, prostate and myeloma.

D. Secondary - Tertiary HPT

1. 2° HPT occurs in renal failure patients on hemodialysis whose serum Ca^{++} is low but whose PTH level remains high. This promotes soft tissue calcification, especially in arteries.

2. 3° HPT is diagnosed when the hemodialysis patient gets a kidney transplant which tries to regulate serum Ca^{++} level but has persistent increased PTH levels causing hypercalcemia.

   a. 3° HPT is usually associated with 4 gland hypertrophy and is treated with either excision of 3 1/2 glands or excision of all glands and reimplantation of 1/2 gland into a forearm muscle.

E. Parathyroid carcinoma

1. Very rare - may not be associated with severely increased Ca^{++}.

2. Suspect it if a palpable tumor mass is present or the parathyroid gland does not easily dissect away from surrounding tissues.

F. Hypoparathyroidism

1. Rare except as complication of thyroid or parathyroid surgery.

2. Treated with calcium and vitamin D supplements.

III. **Adrenal Gland**

A. Anatomy

1. Left side - gland juxtaposes kidney, spleen, pancreas, diaphragm.

   a. Arterial supply from renal artery branches, aortic branches, and phrenic branches.

   b. Main draining vein empties into left renal vein.

2.   Right side - gland juxtaposes kidney, vena cava, liver, diaphragm

     a.   Arterial supply - branch of renal artery, phrenic branch.

     b.   Largest vein is very short and drains into IVC.

B.   Physiology

     1.   Responsible for wide range of mostly cholesterol-derived hormones - catecholamines, aldosterone (mineralocorticoids), glucocorticoids, estrogens, androgens, etc.

C.   Pheochromocytoma

     1.   Metabolically active adenoma (only 10% are malignant) of the adrenal medulla (although 10% are in neuroendocrine rests outside the adrenal gland) that produces catecholamines (1° nor-epinephrine but also epinephrine).

     2.   Associated with MEN II (pituitary, medullary carcinoma of thyroid, pheochromocytoma) and with von Recklinghausen neurofibromatosis but most commonly is an isolated tumor (50-70%). Ten percent are unilateral but in familial cases, 50% are bilateral.

     3.   Usual manifestation is that of sustained high blood pressure (HBP) but the classic manifestations are those of episodic catecholamine release - bursts of HBP, tachycardia, diaphoresis, headaches, weight loss, nausea and vomiting, Raynaud's phenomenon, etc.

     4.   Diagnosis is by detecting VMA and metanephrine levels in urine - localizing tests include CT scanning and/or iodo-cholesterol scans.

     5.   Treatment

          a.   Initial suppression of catecholamine activity - phenoxybenzamine or phentolamine - plus Beta block (propranolol, etc.) if tachycardia develops and simultaneous increasing of intravascular volume.

          b.   Subsequent adrenalectomy.

D.   Primary hyperaldosteronism (Conn's syndrome)

     1.   The most common etiology is a benign adenoma of zona glomerulosa

adrenal gland.

2.   Manifestations include sustained hypertension (usually mild to moderate) with a characteristic hypokalemic metabolic alkalosis and polyuria, polydipsia and muscular weakness.

3.   High serum levels of aldosterone and low levels of serum renin are diagnostic.

4.   Localizing studies include CT scanning or iodo-cholesterol scans.

5.   Treatment consists of excision of the involved adrenal gland, usually through posterior lateral approach.

E.   Cushing's syndrome/disease

1.   Classic Cushing's disease consists of adenoma of anterior pituitary gland secreting cortisol stimulating hormone (ACTH) resulting in stigmata of chronic excess glucocorticoids (60%).

2.   The most common cause of Cushing's syndrome is secondary to iatrogenic administration of glucocorticoids.

    a.   May also result from ectopic source of ACTH (i.e., oatcell carcinoma of lung).

    b.   Adrenal adenomas or carcinomas may occasionally cause Cushing's syndrome (15%).

3.   Manifestations include hypertension, central obesity, purple stria, diabetes mellitus, weakness, amenorrhea, nervousness, irritability, bone pain, osteoporosis, hirsutism, headache, ankle and hand edema, decreased libido in females and feminization of males.

4.   Diagnosis started with urinary and serum cortisol levels. Dexamethasone suppression best may confirm presence of Cushing's syndrome and discriminate the syndrome from the disease.

5.   Localizing efforts include CT scanning and iodo-cholesterol scanning after pituitary adenomas have been ruled out.

6.   Treatment consists of ablation of pituitary if a tumor can be found or bilateral adrenal excision with glucocorticoid and mineral corticoid

replacement.

7. Nelson's syndrome may occur after bilateral adrenalectomy - pituitary enlargement causing visual field loss and hyperpigmentation.

F. Hypoaldosteronism (Addison's disease)

1. Hypoaldosteronism is usually secondary to infectious destruction of the adrenal gland (histoplasmosis) or trauma to the adrenal gland (hemorrhage in patients on anticoagulation or surgical removal).

2. Manifested by unstable blood pressure control and electrolyte abnormalities, becomes a life-threatening problem.

3. Treatment requires glucocorticoid and mineral corticoid replacement.